HAPPIER
No Matter What

Also by Tal Ben-Shahar

Short Cuts to Happiness
The Joy of Leadership
Choose the Life You Want
Happier
Even Happier
Being Happy

HAPPIER
No Matter What

Cultivating Hope, Resilience,
and Purpose in Hard Times

Tal Ben-Shahar, PhD

THE EXPERIMENT

NEW YORK

The Experiment, LLC
220 East 23rd Street, Suite 600
New York, NY 10001-4658
theexperimentpublishing.com

THE EXPERIMENT and its colophon are registered trademarks of The Experiment, LLC. Many of the designations used by manufacturers and sellers to distinguish their products are claimed as trademarks. Where those designations appear in this book and The Experiment was aware of a trademark claim, the designations have been capitalized.

The Experiment's books are available at special discounts when purchased in bulk for premiums and sales promotions as well as for fundraising or educational use. For details, contact us at info@theexperimentpublishing.com.

Library of Congress Cataloging-in-Publication Data

Names: Ben-Shahar, Tal, author.
Title: Happier, no matter what : cultivating hope, resilience, and purpose in hard times / Tal Ben-Shahar, PhD.
Description: New York, NY : The Experiment, LLC, [2021]
Identifiers: LCCN 2021001383 (print) | LCCN 2021001384 (ebook) | ISBN 9781615197910 (hardcover) | ISBN 9781615197927 (ebook)
Subjects: LCSH: Happiness. | Self-actualization (Psychology)
Classification: LCC BF575.H27 B4458 2021 (print) | LCC BF575.H27 (ebook) | DDC 158--dc23
LC record available at https://lccn.loc.gov/2021001383

ISBN 978-1-61519-791-0
Ebook ISBN 978-1-61519-792-7

Jacket design by Beth Bugler
Text design by Jack Dunnington
Author photograph by Judy Rand

Manufactured in the United States of America

First printing May 2021
10 9 8 7 6 5 4 3

To Tami, David, Shirelle, and Eliav—
I love you, no matter what

Contents

Introduction
—
Happier, No Matter What

*To me, the only satisfactory definition of
happiness is wholeness.*

—Helen Keller

"So, Tal, shouldn't we quarantine happiness now?"
my friend asked me. He was only half joking.

We were deep into the coronavirus pandemic
that swept the world. Undeniably, the COVID-19 crisis brought on a particularly intense series of challenges.
Perhaps you got sick, feared becoming ill, or even endured the unimaginable pain of a loved one's death. Perhaps you suffered the loss of your job. Parents struggled
to balance the competing responsibilities of work and
childcare. Families and teachers agonized over whether
it was safe to attend school. And we all felt the malaise
of being isolated from friends and loved ones. For many,
as stresses mounted, the fog of depression set in. Simple
activities that we took for granted and used to turn to for
relaxation vanished overnight, like going out to dinner
or seeing a play, and the joyous celebrations we looked
forward to, like vacations and weddings, were suddenly
canceled. As we masked our faces to protect ourselves
and others from the virus, it even became hard to share
a smile with a stranger while walking down the street.

In the midst of this new reality, what was the relevance of studying happiness? From the time the coronavirus saga started, many people have echoed my friend's sentiment that perhaps we should quarantine happiness, that the science of happiness should be put on hold for a while. They figured, sure, once things are back to normal, we can look at happiness again. But given everything going on in the world right now, shouldn't we press pause?

And my answer to that is no, we shouldn't quarantine happiness. We definitely shouldn't put it on hold! In fact, in challenging times—whatever they may be—studying the science of happiness is more vital and relevant than ever.

Growing from Hardship

We can roughly situate all human experiences along a continuum spanning from negative, through neutral, to positive. For example, pain, suffering, misfortune, and hardship fall on the negative end, while pleasure, joy, fortune, and comfort belong on the positive end. Right in the middle we have the zero point, the "I'm doing OK" point.

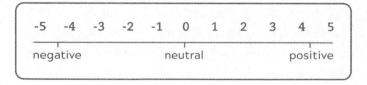

Many people believe that the role of the science of happiness is to deal with anything from neutral to positive. In other words, as long as you're doing OK or better, you can benefit from the research findings in the field. And if you're not doing well—if you're sad or anxious, going through hard times and struggling—well, only psychotherapy or medication can help. Of course, I fully support seeking professional care. Therapy can help whether we're doing fine overall or when our life feels out of control; medication, such as antidepressants or antianxiety drugs, has saved lives, and I would never recommend anyone stop medications without consulting with their physician. But the notion of having to reach "neutral" before one can benefit from the science of happiness is flawed.

The science of happiness is relevant for the entire spectrum of human experiences. Yes, it can certainly help us go from a 3 to a 5, from doing fine to doing really well. But it's even more beneficial when we're at minus 3, or minus 5. It can help us bounce back—and even launch us beyond. Why? Because the science of happiness strengthens our psychological immune system. Needless to say, bolstering your psychological immune system, or your biological immune system for that matter, doesn't mean you won't get sick. It simply means you'll get sick less often, and when you do, you'll recover more promptly. The science of happiness can help you become happier, even if slightly so, no matter where you are along the spectrum. It also equips you to be better able to deal with difficulties and hardships when they arise.

In fact, with a strong psychological immune system, you could go a step beyond resilience. You could become antifragile—what I think of as Resilience 2.0. Antifragile is a concept that was introduced by writer, epistemologist, and statistician Nassim Taleb, a professor at New York University.[1] To understand antifragile, we need to start with resilience, a term taken from engineering. A particular substance or material is considered resilient if it returns to its original form after enduring stress or pressure. Along similar lines, to explain resilience we use the metaphor of a ball dropping and then bouncing back to its original point. According to Taleb, a substance or material is antifragile if, after enduring stress or pressure, it doesn't merely return to its original state, but grows stronger as a result. If a resilient ball bounces back to where it was before, an antifragile ball bounces back higher. More generally, an antifragile system—and that could be an inanimate object or a living entity in the form of a person, a relationship, a group of people, or even a nation—goes through hardship and consequently grows stronger, better, happier.

When Friedrich Nietzsche, the nineteenth-century German philosopher, wrote that "Whatever does not kill me makes me stronger" he was describing antifragility. And, indeed, you can grow from adversity, and experience antifragility, even if you have gone through extreme hardship. Trauma can pull us down or raise us up, leave us weaker or make us stronger.

In fact, research by psychologists Richard Tedeschi and Lawrence Calhoun at the University of North Carolina suggests that people faced with hardships are more likely to experience post-traumatic growth (PTG) than post-traumatic stress disorder (PTSD).[2] Most of us have heard of PTSD, which can include painful consequences like reliving the trauma, anxiety and depression, difficulty concentrating, and trouble sleeping. But there is another potential enduring experience, a beneficial one, and that is PTG. Nothing, unfortunately, can guarantee growth after trauma, however there are certain conditions we can put in place to significantly increase the likelihood of that outcome. As I see it, a central objective of the science of happiness is to help individuals, families, organizations, and communities understand and apply these conditions, and thereby grow from the difficulties associated with the pandemic or any other hardship. There is much that we can do to become more antifragile.

From Research to Me-Search

I wrote this book so that you can have something to anchor you during tumultuous times—ideas that you can hang on to, and most important, experiment with. I'm a psychologist and an academic. In my profession, I draw on research a great deal. However, even more essential than research is me-search. Research is about looking at what other people have done, evaluating their actions, and learning from the result. Me-search is doing the same for the self—looking inside, experimenting with change.

I'm a big fan of biographies. There's much that we can learn from them, especially biographies of people who have done special and extraordinary things. One of my favorites is that of revered Indian leader and activist Mahatma Gandhi. Gandhi's autobiography is subtitled *The Story of My Experiments with Truth*. Notice the language. It's not *My Finding Truth*. It's not *My Discovery of Truth*. It's *My Experiments with Truth*. Throughout his life, standing up for social justice, Gandhi experimented. He tried things. And this is what I would like you to do as you read through this book. Yes, you will learn about a lot of happiness research; yes, you'll find tips for incorporating these ideas in your life. But more than anything, I'd like you to play with these ideas and tips and see how things work for you. Some of the strategies may be highly relevant for you at this point in your journey; some may be relevant for you in the future; and some may not be relevant at all—but it's difficult to know without trying.

Particularly in uncertain times, there's a lot of advice out there on what we should and shouldn't do, whether it's as parents or as employees, whether it's on the personal level or professional. With this book, I hope to distill some evidence-based information so that you can research based on psychological studies and create a bit of order amid the chaos. I want to give you strategies that you can apply and that will help you become happier *now*.

I started to study happiness because of my unhappiness. I'm not sure whether I passed the clinical threshold for depression or anxiety, but I certainly experienced sadness and stress much of the time. That's what led to my interest in positive psychology. Thirty years later, people ask me: "So are you finally happy now?" And my answer to this question is: I don't know. What I do know is that

I am *happier*. As you will learn in this book, the purpose of building antifragility is not to lead you to the happily ever after. I don't believe happily ever after exists. Happiness and unhappiness are not fixed or binary conditions—there isn't a point before which we are unhappy and after which we are happy. Happiness resides on a continuum. I've made a lot of progress over the last thirty years on that continuum, and I certainly hope that five or ten years from now I'll be happier than I am today and that you will be, too. This is why this book is titled *Happier, No Matter What* rather than *Happy, No Matter What*. It's a lifelong journey, one that ends when life ends.

The Myth of Success and Happiness

What exactly is happiness, anyway? Why is it important? And how do we obtain it?

Before we go into definitions, let me share with you a few studies that point to a profound and pervasive misunderstanding about happiness, its role in our lives, and how to get it. Most people believe that the path to happiness is through success. *If only I could achieve my dream—attain this goal, reach that milestone—I would be happy.* Or, following some significant failure, we think, *My dream is over. Everything is ruined. I didn't make it. I'll never be happy now.* According to this formula, success is the cause; happiness is the effect. It turns out, though, that this is wrong—not a little wrong, but *very* wrong.

There are numerous studies that challenge the formula that success leads to happiness. For example, Harvard professor Daniel Gilbert studied college professors at the most important point in their career: just as they were about to hear whether they would receive tenure.[3] When Gilbert asked the professors how they would feel after the tenure decision was made, most predicted that if they received tenure they would enjoy lasting happiness, and if they were turned down, they would be crushed for a long time to come. After all, tenure is considered the holy grail for professors. Often a fifteen-year process, tenure means lifetime employment. It means not being under pressure to publish all the time anymore. It means you get to stay at your university. What actually happened after the decisions were announced? While those professors who received tenure were ecstatic upon hearing the news, and those who were denied tenure were understandably devastated, the major event had little consequences in the long-term for how happy or unhappy they were. In other words, the professors grossly overestimated the impact of a major success—or failure—on their happiness. The event, perceived by most professors as so significant and potentially life changing, led to a temporary high or a temporary low—that's it.

Similar studies have been conducted on lottery winners.[4] How many of us imagine that if we won the lottery, everything would *forever* change for the better? Despite the windfall, it turns out that's not what happens. Lottery winners experience an extreme high when they win, just like the tenured professors. But they go back to where they were before. The winners who had been unhappy usually returned to being unhappy after experiencing a short spike in their happiness levels; no change. The same goes for other big life events, like our wedding day or losing our job: More often than not, we experience a temporary high or temporary low and then go back to where we were before the event on the happiness continuum.

I once informally conducted a poll among my students when I was teaching at Harvard. I had around a thousand students in the class, and I asked them to think back to April 2 of the previous spring, or the years prior. Why April 2? Because that was the day when college acceptance letters used to arrive in the mail (these days it's by email), telling you, *Congratulations, you're in!*, or *We're sorry, our class was very competitive this year.* Given that these students were sitting in my class, of course they had all been accepted. I then said to them: "Please put your hand up if on April 2 you were anywhere between very happy and ecstatic." Just about every hand went up. Then I said, "Please leave your hand up if on April 2 you thought that you would be happy for the rest of your lives." Almost all hands stayed up. Why? Because that's what they were told and consequently believed when they were in high school: Sure, you may be struggling, stressed out, and even miserable now, but if you get into one of your top choices for college, it will forever have been worth it. Then I said, "OK, now leave your hand up if *today* you're happy." I didn't say very happy. I didn't say ecstatic. I just said happy. Most students put their hand down.

The majority of college students around the United States experience stress and are overwhelmed by everything that they have to do.[5] Levels of depression are skyrocketing among teenagers and young adults, and this state of affairs was well underway before the onset of the coronavirus.[6] It's not looking good when it comes to mental health, and yet people continue to believe that success will lead them to the land of happiness. It won't!

Successes do lead you to experiencing highs, while failures lead you to experiencing lows, however these fluctuations are fleeting and in and of themselves are not the building blocks of a happy or unhappy life. Does that mean there isn't a relationship between success and happiness? No. In fact, there's a very strong relationship, but it's the opposite of what most people think. It's not success that leads to happiness; rather it is that *happiness leads to success.*

Why Happiness Matters

Psychologists and organizational scholars consistently demonstrate that if you increase your levels of wellbeing, even by a little bit, you become a great deal more successful.[7] And by successful, I mean not only in the traditional sense of goal achievement—but also in a much broader, multidimensional sense. You'll be more successful as a parent, as a partner, as an employee, as a coach, and as a friend.

By increasing happiness levels even slightly, you become more creative and more innovative, whether in the workplace as an adult, or in school as a child. Productivity and engagement levels, at work and in school, increase significantly in tandem with an increase in wellbeing. Increasing happiness levels makes us kinder and more generous and reduces the likelihood of violence and immoral behavior in general. Our mental and physiological immune systems are linked, and increasing happiness levels fortifies our psychological resilience as well as boosts our physical resilience. Happy people are healthier, better able to ward off disease, and (controlling for all other factors) live longer![8]

And we're not the only ones who benefit when we enjoy an increase in our happiness levels. Happiness improves our relationships, which is even more important when so many of us are remaining in one place, often with the same people, for extended periods of time.[9] But that's not to say that one's being happy eliminates having any conflict at home. You will still experience discontent, you will have disagreements—there may be days when you want to tear your hair out and you can't stand being in such close proximity with the same people. That's OK. That's all part of the "being human" deal. However, even a little boost to wellbeing means you will have fewer relationship challenges, and when you do, you'll be better equipped to deal with them. Moreover, given that happiness is contagious, by increasing your own happiness you help those around you become happier, thus contributing to a happier world—a world that is better, healthier, and more moral.

What Is Happiness?

I'm sure it won't surprise you that happiness has no single agreed-upon definition. In fact, there are probably as many characterizations of happiness as there are human beings, which has led many people, including experts in the field, to argue that happiness is like beauty: You know it when you see it, or experience it. Nevertheless, I maintain that it is important to define happiness for the purpose of understanding it, pursuing it, and attaining it. You may not agree with my definition, and that's fine. I'm not claiming an ultimate truth here. So, whether you use my definition or another, it doesn't matter. What matters is that you think about what happiness is for *you*, and then break it down and understand how you can attain it.

The definition I propose, developed with my colleagues Megan McDonough and Maria Sirois, derives from the work of Helen Keller, who wrote early in the twentieth century, "To me, the only satisfactory definition of happiness is wholeness."[10] Expanding on Keller's words, we define happiness as *whole person wellbeing*. Bringing together the two phrases, *whole person* and *wellbeing*, we offer an even more succinct definition: *Happiness is wholebeing.*

Wouldn't it be great if I could just respond "It's wholebeing!" when people ask me what happiness is? But it's not that simple, for two reasons. First, for this definition to be truly helpful and easy to apply to our lives, we're going to have to dissect "whole person wellbeing" on a more granular level, as we'll soon do. The second reason why this definition is not enough is because of a paradox inherent in our pursuit of happiness.

The Paradox of Happiness

Becoming happier yields many benefits: Your physical immune system strengthens, relationships grow, productivity and creativity increase, and overall performance at work or in school improves. Even without all these benefits, the value of happiness lies in the fact that it simply feels good to feel good. It's in our nature to seek pleasure, avoid pain, and want to experience the flutter of joy rather than the weight of suffering.

But there's a real problem. Studies suggest there is harm in placing too much value on happiness or on becoming happier. UC Berkeley psychologist Iris Mauss (and subsequently others) showed that people for whom happiness is very important—who claim *happiness is a key value of mine*—end up being less happy and feel lonelier in the world.[11] Constantly reminding yourself how important happiness is—and how much you want it—can backfire.

This is the paradox of happiness: The more we value it and therefore want it, the more elusive it is.

If we're trying to become happier, then how do we resolve this paradox? Maybe self-deception? Do we fool ourselves by pretending we don't care, while secretly, deep down, we do? Do we tell ourselves, *I don't want to be happy (wink wink)* . . . ? This gets complicated! Fortunately, there is a solution. We can pursue happiness *indirectly*.

If I wake up in the morning and say to myself, *I want to be happy, I'm going to be happy no matter what!*, I am directly pursuing happiness. This deliberate pursuit to be happy reminds me how important happiness is to me—of how much I value it—and therefore hurts more than it helps. So what does it mean to indirectly pursue happiness? Instead of working at happiness itself, we can pursue the *elements* that lead to happiness. This way our focus is on the value of these elements rather than the value of happiness.

Let's try an analogy: Think about sunlight, vital for life on Earth. What happens if you look *directly* at the sun? It hurts your eyes. It's damaging; you could even go blind. So how can you enjoy seeing the sun? You can look at it *indirectly* and view sunlight through a prism, which breaks it into its components, the colors—making a rainbow. You can then look at, and enjoy, what's right in front of you.

So, too, with happiness. Directly pursuing happiness will lead to unhappiness—this is what Iris Mauss and others found. In contrast, indirectly pursuing happiness—first breaking it down into its elements and then pursuing those elements—is the path to actually becoming happier. In the words of nineteenth-century philosopher John Stuart Mill, "Those only are happy . . . who have their minds fixed on some object other than their own happiness."[12]

Now the important question for us is, what are these other objects that we should focus on? What are the metaphorical colors of the rainbow that make up whole person wellbeing that we *can* pursue, that will indirectly lead us to the light?

Climbing the SPIRE

In developing a way to happiness—combing through the intellectual history of the world and assembling ideas from poets to philosophers, theologians to scientists, economists to psychologists—my colleagues and I have identified five core elements that indirectly lead to happiness: spiritual, physical, intellectual, relational, and

emotional wellbeing.[13] These elements each contribute
to whole person wellbeing and are key to attaining more
happiness. They make up the acronym SPIRE.

Spiritual wellbeing: Are we living mindfully and pur-
posefully? Spiritual wellbeing is about finding a sense
of meaning and purpose. It can certainly be religious,
however, it doesn't have to be. A banker who considers
her work a calling can experience greater spiritual wellbeing than a monk who finds his work devoid of meaning. We also experience spiritual wellbeing when we're
present in the here and now, rather than being distracted
by the then and there. When we're mindful, we elevate
ordinary experiences into extraordinary ones.

Physical wellbeing: Do we take care of our bodies?
This is about the mind-body connection and the impact they have on each other. Physical wellbeing is about
taking care of ourselves through activities like exercise
and through inactivity in the form of rest and recovery.
We nourish our physiological and psychological wellbeing when we eat healthfully and touch lovingly.

Intellectual wellbeing: Are we challenged and curious?
We need to exercise our mind and learn new things.
One of the silver linings of the pandemic was that many
of us, spending more time at home, had more time to engage in intellectual development and growth. Research
shows that people who constantly ask questions and are
eager to learn are not just happier, but are also healthier.
In fact, curiosity contributes to longevity![14]

Relational wellbeing: Do we nurture connections that nurture us? The number one predictor of happiness is quality time we spend with people we care about and who care about us. We are social animals and need to connect, to belong. But it's not just about relationships with others—it's also about our relationship with ourselves. Blaise Pascal, the French philosopher, once said, "All of humanity's problems stem from man's inability to sit quietly in a room alone." Isolation doesn't have to be isolating, and we'll look at how to cultivate healthier and happier relationships even when apart from loved ones.

Emotional wellbeing: Are our feelings both honored and balanced? What do we do with painful emotions when they arise, which they inevitably will? How do we cultivate more pleasurable emotions, like joy, gratitude, and excitement? And how can we reside on higher planes of wellbeing for longer rather than merely enjoy temporary peaks?

These are the five elements that together make up SPIRE, which we'll delve into in this book. *Spire* is a fitting word. One meaning of *spire* is the highest point of a building, like that of a church tower. Happiness is the highest point that we aim for, the star that we aspire to reach. *Spire* also means breath. Happiness gives us breath and increases our energy, engagement, and motivation. Altogether, the elements of SPIRE inspire us to live our best life, a happier life.

What About Financial Wellbeing?

Recently someone said to me, "You need to add a sixth element to SPIRE: financial wellbeing." And he was not the first one to suggest it. When I tell my students about SPIRE, typically someone asks, what about money? This person even went a step further. He noted, "You could call it 'affluential wellbeing,' and then you'll have ASPIRE—you'll still have a nice acronym!" And I did think about it.

The reason I did not add "affluential wellbeing" and go with ASPIRE is because, as I see it, financial wellbeing is already incorporated into SPIRE. The five SPIRE elements are primary characteristics of the person, while financial wellbeing is secondary.

What do philosophers have to say about this hierarchy of primary and secondary characteristics? Aristotle, for example, refers to people as rational animals—that's intellectual wellbeing. Viktor Frankl and the existentialists talk about us as meaning-seeking animals—that's spiritual wellbeing. John Donne wrote "No man is an island"—we are relational animals who need companionship with other people. Emotions, of course, are an essential part of being human, and we don't need Sigmund Freud or David Hume to convince us of that. And when it comes to physical wellbeing, it's about nurturing the animal part of our being, which is most certainly part of our essence (as in rational *animals*, meaning-seeking *animals*, etc.). But there are few if any people who think of humans as financial creatures or as financial animals. Although money can impact our spiritual, physical, intellectual, relational, and emotional lives, it is a tool, rather than a quality intrinsic to the human condition.

This does not mean that financial wellbeing is unimportant. Far from it. Being able to fulfill our basic needs for food, clothing, and housing is vital for us to experience wholebeing. If you are living in poverty and don't have the bare necessities, surely that will affect you and your loved ones. So financial wellbeing has an important role, especially in times of crisis when we are more likely to face financial hardship.

Money does impact happiness up to the point where our basic needs are met; beyond that point, however, having more wealth doesn't contribute much to our wholebeing. What's interesting is that once we have enough to cover our basic needs, what can have a bigger impact on our happiness is not having more money but rather how we use it. Research suggests that spending money on experiences (like an extra vacation), rather than things (like an extra item of clothing), leads to greater happiness.[15] Another thing we can do, perhaps counterintuitively, is to give. As we'll discuss extensively later in this book, when we contribute and help others, we become happier.

Finally, keep in mind that while pursuing the SPIRE elements cannot guarantee financial security, given the relationship between success and happiness, it can certainly help.

Real Change Is Possible

An important step to becoming happier is to recognize that you have the power to increase your happiness. Research by psychologists and neuroscientists—the likes of Richard Davidson, Sonja Lyubomirsky, Jeffrey Schwartz, and Carol Dweck—clearly demonstrates that happiness levels *can and do* change; they are malleable, not fixed.[16] That doesn't mean that you can radically and quickly change your happiness—it's a process that takes time—but small wins, small gains, are certainly possible. If you make a small gain, then another, then even more over a long period of time, you make big gains.

It's a little bit like being on a flight. When sitting on an airplane, watching the small television screen on the back of the seat in front of you, the default channel is a map of the flight path. You might keep your eyes on the little airplane on the map, and it never looks like it's moving. But then you fall asleep (or spend a lot of time trying to), wake up drooling, and look up. What do you see? The plane on the map has moved! You're getting there! Similarly, when it comes to working on your happiness, even if the change is slow and initially imperceptible, over time you will make significant progress.

It's important to mention, though, that no matter how much change you bring about, how much progress you make, you will still encounter hardships, difficulties, and suffering in life. The science of happiness is not a panacea. It is not about magical thinking; nor will it automatically soothe all of your woes. What it *can* do is help you avoid unnecessary suffering. As we'll discuss further in Chapter 5, there are two levels of suffering in adversity. The first is the pain that comes directly from the experience: whether it's concern over our finances, or being upset during a disagreement with a partner, or following a loss. Experiencing this first level of suffering is inevitable. But the second level of suffering comes when we reject the first level, or when we deprive ourselves of basic human needs like exercise and learning and friendship, or when we fail to seize the moment and appreciate all that we have. This book, or any book for that matter, is unlikely to help with the first level of suffering, but it can certainly help with the second.

At the time when I was just finishing up my graduate studies, the economy was tanking. Because part of my PhD was in the business school, I was assigned to help undergrads as they navigated their future careers—with writing their résumés, applying for jobs, and preparing for interviews. One day I was asked to give a talk about the state of the job market. I was blunt with my students. "Look, this is not like last year." The previous year's recruiters had been offering signing bonuses. Now companies were laying off employees. "This year is going to be challenging," I added, "and you're going to have to work harder to find a job." It was then that one student put his hand up and said, "Tal, you are our happiness teacher, you talk to us about optimism, and yet for the past twenty minutes you've been talking nonstop pessimism. Is there any optimistic message that you can share with us?"

There were a few chuckles in the audience and then complete silence. Frankly, I was stumped. Initially, I was going to say that things happen for the best, but before I could open my mouth I realized that I was not fully behind that saying. Things don't always happen for the best. So I said, "I'll get back to you on that." A few days later, I came back to my student with an answer: Things do not necessarily happen for the best, but we can choose to make the best of things that happen.

Whether it's a terrible economy or a devastating pandemic, it's likely not for the best that it's happened. People are anxious, struggling, suffering, even dying as a result. However, whatever the crisis is, it happened. There is nothing we can do about the past, but it is up to us to chart our present and future course. Giving ourselves the permission to be human, exercising regularly, taking time for recovery, being kind, learning from what we're going through, valuing our relationships more, being mindful, appreciating the small things in life—these are all evidence-based practices that we can choose to do to make the best of our situation.

The SPIRE Check-In

At the end of each chapter, you'll find an exercise called The SPIRE Check-In, which will help you assess your personal progress along the way. This is a technique that Maria Sirois, Megan McDonough, and I developed. The SPIRE Check-In is about looking at each element, asking yourself a few simple questions about it, assessing where you are now, and evaluating how you're doing later. It is meant to be a quick snapshot for you of the big picture. Here is an overview of the questions you will find:

Spiritual wellbeing: Do you experience a sense of meaning and purpose in your work? Do you experience a sense of meaning and purpose at home? Are you present? Are you mindful?

Physical wellbeing: How physically active are you? Do you take care of your body? Do you take time for rest and recovery? How do you deal with stress?

Intellectual wellbeing: Are you learning new things? Do you ask enough questions? Do you engage in deep learning? Are you failing enough?

Relational wellbeing: Do you spend quality time with family and friends? Are your relationships deep? Do you take care of yourself? Are you a giver?

Emotional wellbeing: Do you experience pleasurable emotions? Do you embrace painful emotions? Do you take much of what you have in life for granted? Do you appreciate all that you have?

As you go through the SPIRE Check-In and ask yourself each of these questions, grab a pen and paper. The check-in has three steps. The first step is to *ascribe* a score to each of the SPIRE elements. Think about your responses to the questions and determine the degree to which you experience spiritual wellbeing, on a scale of 1 to 10, with 1 being very little or very infrequently, and 10 being very much or very often. To what level, for example, do you experience a sense of meaning? How mindful or distracted are you? Based on your answers, give yourself a score for spiritual wellbeing, and then do the same for physical, intellectual, relational, and emotional wellbeing.

The second step, after you assign a score to each of the SPIRE elements, is to *describe* the reason you gave yourself the score. Why did you give yourself a 6 or a 4 on spiritual wellbeing? Perhaps you find meaning in your family life, but when it comes to work a sense of purpose is largely absent. When it comes to being mindful, maybe you notice *I'm frequently distracted by the news,* and that's why you're not fully present. Maybe you realize you're checking the internet every five minutes. For the five elements of wholebeing, write these reasons down as you describe your predicament.

The final step is to *prescribe*: As concretely and specifically as possible for each of the SPIRE elements, how can you get that score up? Not by 10 points. Not by 5 points. Just by 1 point. What is one thing you can do to find a little bit more meaning in your daily life? How can you be a little bit more mindful with your friends, and so on.

There might be some areas where you're already pleased with your score. If you're satisfied with the 7 you reached for physical wellbeing, you can think about how to maintain it, or you can leave it there and have more time to focus on the areas in which you want to improve. In each chapter, I'll share some ideas for boosting your wellbeing in each realm of SPIRE. This book is about helping you prescribe actions—based on scientific, evidence-based interventions—that can help you increase your score by 1, 2, or maybe even more points in the future.

By assessing each area, we first gain insight into our baseline happiness level. Wherever you are right now, even if it's at 1 or 2 across the board, you can build on that. Remember that it's not about being happy, but about becoming happier. Keep checking in with yourself over the coming weeks, months, and years as you build the antifragility necessary to weather life's ups and downs.

Like a tall building reinforced to withstand an earthquake, SPIRE allows you a support structure for finding happiness even amid life's disasters—and disasters, whether natural or human made, inevitably happen. You may be shaken when the ground suddenly shifts beneath your feet, then shifts some more. But you will not collapse. During a hurricane, you may sway in the fierce winds. But you will not snap. Not only can you emerge from each challenge intact, but you can grow stronger, and happier, than ever.

No matter what.

Chapter 1

—

Spiritual Wellbeing

*The invariable mark of wisdom is to see the
miraculous in the common.*

—Ralph Waldo Emerson

There is a story about a tourist who visited Italy. He comes upon a construction site with workers all around. He approaches one builder and asks him, "What are you doing?" The builder says, "I'm laying bricks."

The tourist walks twenty more yards and sees another builder doing exactly the same thing. He asks that builder, "What are you doing?" The second builder says, "I'm building a wall."

Finally, he sees a third builder on the site, performing the same work as the other two. The tourist asks him, "What are you doing?" The builder looks at him and says, "I'm building a cathedral to the glory of God."

No matter how rote the task or how vast the challenge, our perspective matters a great deal and can make all the difference in terms of our experience.

The first element of the SPIRE of happiness is spiritual wellbeing. Most people associate spirituality with religion or prayer. However, this is by no means a requirement. While spirituality can certainly be experienced in a synagogue, a church, a mosque, or a temple, we can also find it in our day-to-day lives. We can experience spirituality in two ways: when we're feeling a sense of meaning and purpose in what we're doing, and when we're fully present and focused in the moment.

There's an important distinction we need to make when we talk about spirituality. Viktor Frankl, in his book *Man's Search for Meaning*, distinguishes between "the meaning *of* life" and "meaning *in* life." The meaning of life might encompass questions like *Why am I here? What is the purpose of it all? What is life all about?* Many people seek these answers in religion, or perhaps in a noble mission for the greater good, such as overcoming poverty or ending global warming. It's often difficult to find the meaning of life—and it can be daunting to wrestle with the concept, especially during hard times when we are simply trying to get through the day. In contrast, it's easier to find meaning *in* life: in the ordinary things that we do routinely, in the present moment, in our daily activities at home or work. And it's the meaning in life that we'll primarily explore as a way to experience spiritual well-being—through that concept, we'll open up the possibility of a genuinely happier life, even in challenging times.

The Power of Purpose

How do you feel about what you do these days? What motivates you?

Research can help us understand how we view our own work. At the University of Michigan, organizational psychologists Amy Wrzesniewski and Jane Dutton conducted an eye-opening study on purpose.[1] They identified that people perceive their work in one of three distinct ways.

There are people who mostly see their work as a job—a chore you do solely out of necessity because you need the paycheck. A job is something you have little choice about doing. If you fall into this category, you experience a sense of obligation. What do you look forward to when you're in a job? Perhaps the end of the shift, the end of the week, a long-awaited vacation, or the day when you can finally retire.

Then there are people who primarily see their work as a career: climbing the organizational ladder. For them, it's all about being in the rat race and getting ahead. Seeing your work as a career is future- and reward-oriented. You're motivated to work because you want to advance: You're looking forward to the raise, the bonus, the promotion.

And then there are people who view their work as a calling. Seeing your work as a calling is experiencing it as purposeful. It's about looking forward to more work because you genuinely care about it, enjoy it, and have a passion for doing it beyond a sense of duty or the need for a paycheck. Your work has significance for you. It's meaningful.

Most of us experience all three perspectives, at different times. We have days when our work is a grind, we have days when we're focused on advancement, and we have days when we truly love what we do. The question is, which is the predominant mindset? How do you feel about your work in general?

Consider which one of these statements you most identify with:

- I primarily see my work as a job. I don't enjoy it, but I have to do it.

- I primarily see my work as a career. I'm all about making progress and succeeding.

- I primarily see my work as a calling. I am passionate about what I do and see it as meaningful.

Wrzesniewski and Dutton went to various workplaces and studied their employees, identifying and grouping them by these mindsets. In one study, they visited hospitals and spoke to employees across different roles and positions. The first group they looked at were the janitors, responsible for sweeping the floors, cleaning the toilets, and changing the bedsheets, day in and day out. Among the janitors, they found those who saw their work as a job. *I do it because I have no choice, I need to make money to live on. I can't wait for the end of my shift.* Then there were janitors performing the very same tasks who saw their work as a career. For them it was about working to get to the next level, advancing to a more senior role with better pay. And then there were janitors in those very same hospitals, sweeping the floors, cleaning the toilets, changing the bedsheets, who viewed their work as part of something important: They were contributing to the work of the doctors and nurses and to the healing of patients.

Not surprisingly, the third group of janitors, who viewed their work as meaningful, also acted differently.

They were by and large more generous and helpful, more friendly and more likely to talk with patients about how they were doing. Naturally, even this group of janitors had their job days, when they just wanted to get home, or their career days when their primary concern was moving up and making more money. But overall, they experienced their day-to-day as a calling.

Next, Wrzesniewski and Dutton talked to the doctors and found that they could also be grouped according to these three perspectives. There were doctors for whom work was a chore. For this group, it was *Let this week be over. I've been doing this for twenty years, and I've had enough.* There were doctors who went through tasks as stepping-stones to becoming the head of their ward, or the chief of the department. *When do I get that raise? How about that promotion?* And then there were the passionate doctors for whom work was a vocation. *This is what I'm supposed to do with my life.* Although the researchers found a greater percentage of doctors than janitors with the calling perspective, there were still doctors who primarily viewed their work as a job or career. The same pattern was discovered by Wrzesniewski and Dutton, and other researchers, in numerous other professions—among engineers, schoolteachers, bankers, and hairdressers. It turns out that the dominant perspective in your life makes all the difference in terms of your overall wellbeing, as well as how you end up doing in that work in the long run.

My business partner, Angus Ridgway, has a brother-in-law who is a cardiologist and whose specialty is implanting pacemakers. After implantation, every few years he takes out the pacemaker, replaces the battery, and puts it back in. Angus was having lunch with his brother-in-law one day and said, "I finally figured out what you do for a living." His brother-in-law replied, "Oh really? What do I do for a living?" and Angus, always the one to find humor in situations, said, "You change batteries."

His brother-in-law looked at him intently and said, "Angus, you're right. Some days I change batteries. Other days I save lives." Herein lies the distinction.

I once witnessed a calling mindset in what I considered unlikely circumstances: trying to get a mortgage. A few years ago, my wife and I found our dream home. When we realized how much it would cost, it threatened to become a nightmare. But it was a home that we really loved and wanted, so we decided to go for it.

The following day we went to the bank to ask for a mortgage. We met the mortgage officer, and the minute I saw her I noticed something peculiar about her: She was unusually cheerful. We sat down and she went over a mind-numbing number of Excel sheets with us, yet she was remarkably upbeat with every click of the mouse. "This is 4.1 percent interest! This is 3.9 percent! This is a 15-year loan, this is a 30-year loan!"

Eventually, we were approved for a mortgage. When we came back a few weeks later to sign all the paperwork—not a short process—the loan officer was again smiling and chipper throughout the entire forty-minute session. At the end of the meeting, I said to her, "You like your work, don't you?" And she responded, "I love my work." I said, "Really? Why?" to which she replied: "It's because every day I get to help people fulfill their dreams." A few seconds went by, she looked at us, smiled, and then added: "Today, I am going to do the same for you." And so she did. My wife and I are still grateful to her for helping us realize our dream.

There are probably hundreds of thousands of mortgage officers all around the world. I could be wrong—and maybe it's just that spreadsheets make my eyes glaze over—but I'd wager that those who primarily see their work as a calling are not the majority. But they exist, and that fact changes the question from "Is it possible to find a calling?" to "*How* is it possible to find a calling?"

The calling mindset doesn't just apply to the workplace. Let's say you have little kids at home. Six o'clock in the evening comes, and it's time to start the dinner-to-bedtime routine. Let's look at three scenarios.

1. At six PM you cringe and say to yourself, *Oh no, not again!* But of course, you have to take care of your children. It's your obligation. Reluctantly, you cook, sit down, and have dinner. The kids don't behave so well, but somehow you get through dinner and then start the bath routine. Water gets splashed all over the floor—one more thing to clean up. The kids brush their teeth. Once in bed they want a story, and they insist you read them the same book as the night before, *The Little Engine That Could*. The train goes up that same mountain again. They're excited about it, so you read it to them. After all, it's your responsibility, right? Finally, they fall asleep. Parenting as a job!

2. **Six PM comes, and it's time to make your kids dinner.** You decide you'd better prepare some vegetables with dinner, and you beg your kids to eat them. You want them to grow up to be healthy adults, after all. You then take them through the bath time and teeth-brushing routines and make sure they scrub; it's important to create good hygiene habits. You've recently come across research that says kids who are read to are more successful later in life, so you make sure to read them a book, even if it's the same story you read to them last night. You're nearly falling asleep yourself, but you do it because it matters for their future. Parenting as a career!

3. **Six PM comes.** As you sit with your family at the dinner table, the kids are goofing off as usual. But you pause your fork for a moment, look around, and observe, *What a privilege. What a privilege it is to be spending time with the most important people in my life. Look at how my children are growing up. Look at them talking and enjoying themselves.* At bath time, the kids are having fun splashing, and you joke, play games, and make funny faces together. They brush their teeth and go to bed. In bed, they want the same story again. As you read it you're struck by how excited your kids are, as if they're hearing this story of the train going up the hill for the first time. And when you see the joy in their eyes, you feel gratitude for these precious little beings that you get to spend time with. They go to sleep. Parenting as a calling!

My wife and I have three kids. Every night of parenting is a calling for us, right? Most certainly not! It isn't for any parent. We all have our challenges, the kids push our buttons, and sometimes, it's *Just let the day be over, please!* While you don't have to be all-in 24/7 on the wonders of parenting, can you make more space for that spiritual experience? Can you increase the time each day, even by just a bit, that you pause to notice and connect to that which is meaningful?

Whatever your responsibilities, whether at home or at work, you have significant control over how you perceive them. Finding meaning in your activities can make all the difference in terms of how you go through your days, your weeks, your life. In the words of Wrzesniewski and Dutton, "Even in the most restricted and routine jobs, employees can exert some influence on what is the essence of their work."[2] Now change "routine jobs" to "routine life." This phrase has described our existence more than ever as we live through a pandemic. We wake up, turn on the coffee maker, answer email, log in to a meeting on Zoom. We barely leave the house to shop. We don't have spontaneous nights out. We don't travel. The days blend together: We live an ultra-routine life. But despite the often-accompanying feelings of social isolation, uncertainty, and anxiety, we can still experience more of our time as a calling. We can exert some influence on the essence of our life. How? By identifying the significance in our day-to-day activities.

Again, this is not about the broader meaning *of* life—that's a discussion for another time. It's about a simple change you can make to connect with the meaning *in* life. What is that one change for you?

A Calling Description

Try this exercise: Choose a routine task and write down the actions you do to complete it—a "job description" of sorts. For me, it might be preparing a lecture for class. *I sit in front of my computer, do some reading, and then write up an outline for the presentation. After going over the notes a few times, I deliver the lecture to my students. After class, I analyze how the lecture went.* Then, try reframing the same routine task as a "calling description"—focusing on the significance of each step. Why do you do it? If you get stuck, reflect on it like you're finishing these sentences:

"This is important to me because _____."

"I'm passionate about _____."

"I help others by _____."

Reflecting on how I prepare for class from the perspective of these questions, here's what I do: *I start the process by engaging with fascinating content from the world's greatest thinkers. I get to integrate the material into a coherent outline, which helps me to understand it, and myself, better. Then, I get to share what I care so much about with other people, helping them become happier. After a lecture, I go back and ask myself, what did I learn from the questions that were asked in class? What can I build on? How can I continue to grow as a teacher and make a difference in people's lives?*

This exercise can be especially helpful to re-center yourself when you're stuck in the job doldrums, or when you're hitting roadblock after roadblock. Back in the nineteenth century Friedrich Nietzsche wrote that "He who has a why to live for can bear almost any how." When there is a sense of meaning and purpose in what we do,

the path to overcoming difficulties becomes less daunting. Very often, connecting with your purpose is what
makes the difference between fragility and antifragility:
between breaking down and growing stronger, between
despair and optimism.

Adam Grant, a professor of psychology at Wharton,
conducted research on telemarketers whose job it was to
fundraise for a university.[3] "Hello, this is John from your
alma mater. Can you donate?" What word do you think
these solicitors hear most often? Not surprisingly, it's *no*. If
they're lucky, it's "No, thank you, I've already donated."
Frequently, it's "Don't call this number again" or "Leave
me alone" in stronger language. They repeat this demor-
alizing conversation dozens of times a day.

Grant randomly divided the university fundraisers
into two groups. For the first group, it was business as
usual: They continued to just make calls all day. But he
pulled the second group away from their work for fifteen
minutes—that's all. During that fifteen-minute break, he
had them talk with a student from their university who
was on financial aid—a student who was the beneficiary
of their work as a fundraiser. Many students could not
have attended college without financial assistance. Those
students told the fundraisers, "Thank you for what you
do." For fifteen minutes, they expressed gratitude: talking
about what an amazing time they were having in college,
what a privilege it was to be at this university, and how
grateful they were for the money raised for their education. Afterward, the fundraisers went back to the phones.

The result of that brief intervention? Grant discovered
that the fundraisers found their work more meaningful.

They had more energy and were more engaged. Amazingly, they were more successful, too: They raised between 250 and 400 percent more money compared to the control group, just because they were reminded of how important their work was. All it took was a small shift in perspective.

Now, take a moment or two to step back and recognize the true value and intention of what *you* do, whether it is helping your kids with their homework, washing the dishes by yourself, going over the bills with your partner, caring for an aging parent, negotiating a deal with a client, or pushing through a difficult assignment at work. It doesn't take much, just a few minutes of awareness—and that can make all the difference.

Mindfulness

We can also experience spirituality through mindfulness meditation—we can practice being aware in the moment, free from distraction. Mindfulness is present-moment awareness, ideally without judgment. It can be awareness of breath, another physical sensation, an object, an activity, or anything else.

Cultural traditions and writings that center on mindfulness meditation go back thousands of years. There are the Tibetan Book of the Dead, the sutras of the Indian thinker Patanjali, the Tao teachings from China, and the spiritual exercises of Philo of Alexandria, to name a few. In each of these traditions and many others, there is much discussion on the importance of being fully present in the here and now. Today, we have evidence for what adherents of these traditions have long known: Mindfulness has many benefits for wellbeing.

Most of our dark moments are a result of our inability to be present. The more present we are, the more enlightened moments we experience. Vietnamese Buddhist monk Thich Nhat Hanh says, "If we're living in the past we're open to depression; in the future we're open to anxiety; only in the present are we open."[4] Those who regularly practice mindfulness report feeling calmer and more content. Moreover, there's neuroscientific evidence that meditation has a discernable impact on the structure of the brain itself.

Until the latter part of the twentieth century, most psychologists and neurologists believed that the brain was essentially fixed, its neural makeup and structure predetermined by genes and early childhood experiences. But more recently, with the help of modern technology, breakthrough research on neuroplasticity and neurogenesis has clearly demonstrated that our brain can and does change.[5] In fact, our brain continues to change throughout our lives, from the moment we're born until the day we die. And it turns out that one of the most effective ways of sculpting our brain, of altering our neural circuitry to promote overall wellbeing, is mindfulness meditation.[6] Thanks to EEG, fMRI, and other scanning technology, we know that the brain of a dedicated meditator—who meditates regularly and extensively—looks radically different from a non-meditator's. It's a happier brain.

There are many studies on the importance of mindfulness meditation. One study done jointly by Jon Kabat-Zinn, founder of the Stress Reduction Clinic at the University of Massachusetts Medical Center, and Richard Davidson, director of the Center for Healthy Minds at the University of Wisconsin–Madison, laid out the essential benefits.[7] Kabat-Zinn and Davidson invited people to participate in an eight-week intervention, the Mindfulness-Based Stress Reduction Program. The program consisted of a weekly three-hour class on meditation, followed by homework, which was to meditate on one's own for forty-five minutes every day. At the end of the eight weeks, the researchers compared the moods of those who completed the course to prospective students who had an interest in learning meditation but hadn't yet started the course. After comparing the two groups, they found that the students who went through the eight-week meditation course experienced more positive moods, less anxiety, and were more social and outgoing. The course had a real impact on happiness.

The findings were not only based on self-reports. The researchers also employed physiological measures, and what they found was remarkable. Specifically, they measured neural activation in the prefrontal cortex, the part of the brain responsible for complex emotional, cognitive, and behavioral functions. People who have more neural activation on the left side tend to be happier, while people who have more activation on the right side tend to be more depressed. A high left-to-right ratio goes hand in hand with higher susceptibility to pleasurable emotions, resilience to painful emotions, and a greater ability to remain calm. The researchers found that as a result of the eight-week program, the brain of participants changed significantly: The left side of the prefrontal cortex became more active relative to the right side. While their brains weren't as "positive," so to speak, as those who had spent years upon years meditating, in as little as two months there was already a significant change. They actually became happier, and brain imaging clearly showed the progress that they made.

As part of the study, the researchers injected participants as well as the control group with cold bacteria and measured their immune responses. Amazingly, those who went through the meditation program produced more antibodies to the bacteria. In other words, their immune system strengthened and they became more resilient, physically as well as psychologically. In merely eight weeks of practicing mindfulness meditation, they became healthier and happier.

What Is Meditation?

The word *gom* is Tibetan for meditation and literally means "to become familiar with." So meditation is about becoming familiar with something. We can meditate on our breath, observing it and getting to know it; we can get to know physical sensations while holding a yoga posture; we can also meditate on the nature of an emotion, exploring whatever it is that we're feeling.[8]

We're often consumed by the many tasks and obligations vying for our attention, by worries about the future circling overhead, by the "should've done"s tugging at our sleeve. Buddhists refer to the distracted mind as the "monkey mind," swinging from vine to vine, jumping around and not stopping for a split second. The goal of meditation is to rest the monkey mind, to help it stop jumping around so much, because when we rest it, we are more likely to see clearly— to become familiar with whatever it is that we're observing.

There is an African fable about a hippopotamus who, while crossing a river, lost one of his eyes. Frantically, the hippopotamus began to look for it. He looked behind him, in front of him, on both sides, underneath, but to no avail. From the bank of the river, the river birds and other animals suggested that the hippopotamus take some time off to rest and recover, but he refused, fearing that he would never find his eye. And so he continued desperately searching without success, until he was so tired that he had to take a break. As soon as he stopped moving and calmed down, the river calmed down as well. The mud he had stirred up sank to the bottom, and the water became still and transparent. And there, resting on the bottom of the river, he saw his eye. Similarly, in order to see an object clearly and to become familiar with it—whether it's our mind or a word or an emotion—we need to stop, rest, and allow the murky water to settle before the object can emerge.

There are four main guidelines to a meditation practice. Not every practitioner or scholar will agree with me here, but I have found these to be the most common and most important ones.[9] They are:

1. **Allow the mind to rest on a single object.** Pay attention to one thing, be it your breath, your posture, a feeling, a sound, an object, or anything else within or without.

2. **Return to focus.** The key to mindfulness meditation is not maintaining focus but returning to focus. In other words, rather than the continuous and uninterrupted act of focusing, what matters is catching your mind when it wanders off and reestablishing focus.

3. **Breathe slowly, gently, and deeply.** The most health-enhancing, wholesome breath is what's called belly breath, where we take in air and fill our lungs until we see our belly rising and falling.

4. **Accept that there is no good or bad meditation.** This is about suspending judgment, accepting the experience as is; judging a practice, or ourselves, as good or bad goes against the very spirit of mindfulness meditation. For example, whether we held our focus for 98 percent of our time or whether our mind constantly wandered doesn't matter. And if we feel better as a result of the practice, or worse, or if it made absolutely no difference, doesn't matter either.

The key to reaping the many benefits of meditation is repetition. UCLA psychiatrist Daniel Siegel writes: "Just as people practice daily dental hygiene by brushing their teeth, mindfulness meditation is a form of brain hygiene—it cleans out and strengthens the synaptic connections in the brain."[10] And just as you start and end your day with brushing your teeth, you can start or end your days by meditating.

As little as three to five minutes a day of meditation, practiced consistently, can have a positive impact on your overall wellbeing. And if you do twenty to thirty minutes, even better. The short meditation sessions are analogous to a quick shower; the longer sessions can be compared to a luxuriating bath. Both are cleansing.

An Easy Way to Meditate

If you'd like to experience a short meditation, start here.

Go to a quiet place where you are alone. Find a comfortable position. You can be sitting down or lying on your back, whatever feels right for you. You can do this with your eyes closed or open; it doesn't matter.

As you are in this comfortable position, lengthen your spine from your tailbone all the way up to your neck. Keep your spine straight, but not strained.

Breathe in and out through your nose, if possible. If not, breathing through your mouth is perfectly fine.

Now allow your attention to rest on the breath going in through your nose or mouth and filling up your belly, and then leaving your belly and out through your mouth or nose. Continue to breathe in slowly and deeply and then breathe out slowly and gently. Your belly goes up with each inhalation and down with each exhalation.

Just as it is natural to breathe, it is also natural that the mind wanders. When it does, gently bring it back to the breath, focusing on the air going in and out. You have nothing to do and nowhere to go. You are just being with the breath, with the present. If your mind strays, gently, with acceptance, bring it back to your belly going up and down. Continue for as long as you like, and when you're ready to end the session, gently open your eyes.

This is just a simple experience of meditation. There are thousands of guided meditations online, and I urge you to experiment with different ones. You're sure to find some that you connect to, and that in turn connect you to the present moment.

Finding the Sacred in the Mundane

Let's revisit the study by Jon Kabat-Zinn and Richard Davidson for a moment. At the end of the eight-week program, researchers asked participants for how long they actually meditated in between sessions. Remember, the participants were asked to meditate for forty-five minutes every day. What the researchers found, as expected, was that not everyone complied with the homework assignment. Some students indeed meditated for forty-five minutes a day. But then there were students who only meditated for twenty minutes a day, or just twice a week. The fascinating thing was that it didn't make a difference! Those who meditated only twice a week enjoyed all the same benefits—psychological and physiological—as those who meditated daily over those eight weeks.

Why is it that participants gain benefits even if they do not do their homework and meditate? The answer in all likelihood lies in the fact that participants were reminded to be mindful, and were mindful whether or not they stopped to meditate. You see, we can be mindful anywhere and anytime—right now, of the words we read or the breath we're taking, or while participating in a meeting or while doing the laundry. In the words of Dr. Elisha Goldstein, author of *The Now Effect*: "Mindfulness is basically just being aware, and can be practiced both informally and formally . . . When you're practicing it informally, that means that you're simply attempting to be more aware in everything that you do—and that mentality can be infused into pretty much anything.

But the formal practice of mindfulness is mindfulness meditation."[11]

It seems, then, that the benefits of mindfulness come, whether we do it formally—sitting down for however long and focusing on the breath going in and out—or informally—carrying out any activity while being present to it and reminding ourselves to return to presence when our mind wanders. Participants in the eight-week program were reminded weekly how important it is to be present, and as a result they were mindful more often, and it didn't matter whether they were formally mindful for the forty-five minutes a day, or informally mindful while engaging in other daily activities.

By being mindful, we can turn the mundane into the sacred, the ordinary into the extraordinary—and hence increase our spiritual wellbeing. We can do that when we're risking our life for freedom or while conversing with our friend over dinner, praying at a temple or creating an Excel spreadsheet at work. In the words of Thich Nhat Hanh, "At any moment, you have a choice, that either leads you closer to your spirit or further away from it."[12]

Becoming Aware (Informally)

To my mind, the most important teaching in the literature on mindfulness is that leading a spiritual life is not to be found in some faraway destination, but rather right here and right now. Rather than searching for the far-off and illusive "happily ever after," we can find wholesome moments spread throughout our tumultuous journey. These moments are valuable—first, because they are joyful in themselves, and second, because they provide us with the fuel we need to power through life's misadventures.

You can enjoy present-moment awareness formally, as you close your eyes and focus on your breath going in and out; or while standing in a yoga posture (an asana) and focusing on your physical sensations. You can also experience present-moment awareness—and its benefits—informally, during basically any activity during the day. Whether eating, doing chores, folding laundry, taking a walk, writing an email, or playing fetch with your dog, you can practice being fully present while doing it. In the words of American author Henry Miller, "The moment one gives close attention to anything, even a blade of grass, it becomes a mysterious, awesome, indescribably magnified world in itself."[13] Miller is describing how, by being mindful, we can infuse the world and our life with spirit. Here are some suggestions for how to incorporate more mindfulness, and therefore spiritual wellbeing, into your daily life.

Listen
Our instinct in a conversation can be to mentally jump ahead to what *we* want to talk about, whether it's because we think we know what the other person is about to say or we think we know what the other person needs to hear. Other times, it's all too easy to tune out. We let our mind wander to other things, like the next item on our to-do list. As we catch up with a friend on the phone, we might be idly scrolling through an article or social media at the same time. But how often do we truly stop what we are

doing, and just listen? Do we let ourselves hear, be open to, and be thoughtful about, the other person's words?

There's a lot of research on the benefits of simply listening—to both the listener and the person being listened to.[14] By paying attention, the people listening enjoy the benefits of an informal mindfulness practice. Children who are listened to grow up to be more positive, more confident adults. Employees who are listened to by their superiors are less likely to leave their company and more likely to give their all at work. Not surprisingly, spouses who listen to each other have healthier relationships and are more likely to stay together. In fact, the foundation of any deep relationship—with your child, partner, best friend, parent, or colleague—is listening.[15]

Equally important for wholebeing is listening to yourself, which you can do by keeping a journal and journeying inward, mindfully exploring your own thoughts, heartfully engaging with your desires. Just writing and experiencing, without judgment or criticism, can be liberating while at the same time help you connect to yourself and to the world.[16]

Disconnect to Connect

The crazy-busy pace of modern life coupled with the increasing need for multitasking makes distraction—rather than focus—the norm. A simple way to reverse this tide is to take a break from your phone and your laptop. Ongoing and erratic stimulations in the form of an incoming email, a ringing phone, a flashing screen, or background noise lead us to gradually lose our ability and inclination to be present and focused. Silencing your phone, having a "technology-free" time of day or place in your home, and refraining from multitasking are all ways of facilitating practicing mindfulness informally.

Savor

Eating is another ordinary activity through which we can choose to experience the benefits of mindfulness. A few years ago I participated in a mindfulness workshop, and one of our exercises was to eat a raisin. You can easily do this at home, too. I don't mean just pop it into your mouth and swallow it in a second, but truly *eat a raisin*. First, pick up just one raisin and look at it. Notice the texture, the colors. A raisin is not just brown; there are different colors that emerge—purple, orange, black—depending on where the light shines on it. Smell the raisin. Familiarize yourself with its distinct, sweet scent. Now you can put the raisin in your mouth, but don't chew it. Roll the raisin around on your tongue and feel it. Then, take a bite of it, just one bite. What do you notice?

We have to be present in order to observe all the different tastes that emerge from that one raisin. It can take fifteen minutes or more to eat a single raisin! Now, I don't recommend doing this entire exercise every time you take a bite of something. But I do recommend trying it a few times this week, and beyond that, making time to savor your food in general. Perhaps you can make it a ritual to take ten minutes each day or even just once a week to experience a food or a meal with all your senses. Really focus on the amazing textures, scents, and tastes that make the food unique and special.

Presence Is a Gift

In 1999, a leading scholar in the field of positive psychology, Mihaly Csikszentmihalyi, asked a simple question: "If we are so rich, why aren't we happy?"[17] Csikszentmihalyi was alluding to the research demonstrating that even though our generation is wealthier than previous ones, we are not happier for it. In fact, while levels of material prosperity are on the rise, so are levels of depression and anxiety. There are various reasons for this unfortunate situation that span the entire SPIRE rainbow—from the fact that people are spending more time sitting down rather than moving, to the increase of virtual relationships and the decrease of real connections. With all that, one of the main reasons for the declining levels of mental health in both children and adults is the rising levels of distraction from the present moment. The antidote to this distraction is a commitment to engaging with whatever it is that is inside or in front of us now.

Psychotherapist Tara Bennett-Goleman, in her wonderful book *Emotional Alchemy*, provides an eloquent answer to Csikszentmihalyi's question, explaining why our growing material wealth is not translating into an increase in levels of happiness—and what we can do to change that:

> The richest banquet, the most exotic travel, the most interesting, attractive lover, the finest home—all of these experiences can seem somehow unrewarding and empty if we don't really attend to them fully—if our minds are elsewhere, preoccupied with disturbing thoughts. By the same token, the simplest of life's pleasures—eating a piece of fresh-baked bread, seeing a

work of art, spending moments with a loved one—can be amply rich if we bring a full attention to them. The remedy to dissatisfaction is inside us, in our minds, not in groping for new and different outer sources of satisfaction.[18]

Bennett-Goleman is pointing to the countless opportunities we have for informal mindfulness and how we can find spiritual wellbeing in just about everything that we do, merely by being present to the experience. And yet, most of the time, most people are disengaged and miss out on the potential for spiritual wellbeing. Fortunately, the opportunities for finding more meaning are ubiquitous and pervasive. Albert Einstein purportedly once said, "There are only two ways to live your life. One is as though nothing is a miracle. The other is as though everything is a miracle." As you mindfully engage with life—whether on the yoga mat, while taking a walk outside alone, or as you chat with a friend—everything becomes a miracle, a spiritual experience.

At one time or another we have all experienced something in our day-to-day life as a miracle. Think back to a time when you were able to see beyond the ordinary and into the extraordinary, to experience life as the against-all-odds wonder that it is. You may have been struck by it when you read a poignant passage in a book that captured you or listened to a beautiful piece of music that moved you. Perhaps you experienced the extraordinary while feeling the wind brush your skin during a walk across the park or while feeling the satisfaction of finally completing a challenging project at work. You may have felt it while watching a baby learn to walk or a harvest moon rise in the sky. The common element to all these experiences is one of being mindful rather than mindless. You were absorbed in the activity, fully engaged, living in the now.

It is hardly a coincidence that the word for this moment is *present*: This moment, as every moment, has the potential to be a gift.

Spiritual Wellbeing

Go through the three steps of the SPIRE Check-In—ascribe, describe, and prescribe—focusing on spiritual wellbeing. Begin by reflecting on the following questions:

Do you experience a sense of meaning and purpose in your work?

Do you experience a sense of meaning and purpose at home?

Are you present?

Are you mindful?

Based on your reflections, determine the degree to which you experience spiritual wellbeing and then *ascribe* a score from 1 to 10, with 1 being very little or very infrequently, and 10 being very much or very often. After ascribing a score, *describe* in writing why you gave yourself that score. Then, *prescribe* a way to increase your score by just 1 point at first. Examples may include writing a "calling description," pausing what you're doing twice a day to connect with your purpose, starting a five-minute daily mindfulness practice, or committing yourself to doing only one thing at a time for an hour or two a day. Keep checking in with yourself once a week.

Chapter 2

—

Physical Wellbeing

Sometimes your joy is the source of your smile, but
sometimes your smile can be the source of your joy.
—Thich Nhat Hanh

The study of happiness is always relevant, no matter what you're going through. It obviously helps in good times, but it's no less important in getting us through difficult times. It contributes to our resilience and helps us become antifragile; in other words, it strengthens us when we're facing a challenge.

As I write this in 2020, in the midst of shutdowns resulting from the pandemic, many of us have experienced an incredibly challenging year and have responded in different ways. For example, I know people who actually started off doing well—for them, at first, social distancing and staying home was a good way to shift into a lower gear, spend more time with their loved ones, and take more time to appreciate what they have, rather than take it for granted. They were doing fantastic. But with almost no exceptions, at some point they each experienced a downturn in their mood and overall wellbeing. It hit them that this was not a vacation, but a new normal of sorts, and that took the wind from their sails. Others who started off very anxious and uncertain eased into their reality and began to feel better. And then there are others—likely the majority—who were constantly going through ups and downs. They had cheerful days and terrible days; calm periods and frantic ones. But the common denominator among most everyone was a feeling of being overwhelmed and stressed in unprecedented ways.

There's still cause for optimism: By taking simple steps to improve your physical health, you can make strides in your resilience and happiness. This chapter will focus on the mind-body connection, on how psychology and physiology are part of one interconnected system. Among the characteristics of this system that we'll explore is how physical toughness generates mental toughness, and how stress—when properly understood and handled—can contribute to our wellbeing rather than undermine it.

The Mind and Body Are One

The first step to fulfilling our potential for physical wellbeing is to recognize the inseparable connection between mind and body. What gets in the way, however, is a widespread belief, known as dualism, that the mind and body are distinct entities.[1]

Why is the dualistic perspective problematic? MIT systems scientist Peter Senge wrote, "Dividing an elephant in half does not produce two small elephants." He explains, "Living systems have integrity . . . their character depends on the whole."[2] In the same way, dividing a human being into two—into a mind and a body—does not produce two small human beings or two viable entities that we can cultivate and grow. It is an artificial separation. If we want to effect change, we need to look at the whole person. Remember, happiness is whole person wellbeing.

The unity of mind and body manifests itself in various ways. For example, your thoughts and emotions influence your body—from its posture to its performance—while in turn your movements can affect your mindset and heartset. Research on the "facial feedback hypothesis" highlights this connection: Putting on a smile or frown, a kind face or an angry face, generates the emotion that we associate with the face.[3] When subjects imitated the face of an angry person, their heart rate and skin temperature increased, and they started to think angry thoughts.

It's not just our face, but our entire body that can be used to change our mood. Psychologist Sara Snodgrass of Florida Atlantic University asked one group of study participants to walk for three minutes in a certain manner: long strides, arms swinging, and looking up. This walk is the external manifestation of a confident, upbeat mood. She asked a second group of participants to shuffle, take small steps, and look down. This walk is associated with a more brooding, dejected mood. The result? The first group was more upbeat following their three minutes of the "happy" walk. This experiment and many others help explain why we usually feel good, or at least better, after we dance or go for a run. Beyond the physiological impact of exercise, which we'll discuss later in the chapter, the very posture we assume while dancing or running is beneficial for our emotional state.[4]

Here's another experiment that dramatically underscores the connection between mind and body.[5] Scientists at the Cleveland Clinic divided participants into four groups and had them do exercises for fifteen minutes per day, five days a week, for twelve weeks. The first group was taught "mental contractions" of their little finger—they were to imagine exercising the finger without moving it. The second group used their imagination to exercise their biceps, envisioning bending their elbow. The third group actually exercised their finger, contracting it with physical resistance. The fourth group, the control group, did nothing. The results? The control group did not get any stronger, which is no surprise. Also, predictably, the third group that physically exercised their finger increased their finger strength by 53 percent. The surprising result is that the first group—that only mentally exercised—increased their finger strength by 35 percent. Without lifting a finger! The group that imagined themselves exercising their biceps increased their strength by 13.5 percent. Mind and body are connected, part of the same whole, and to fulfill our potential for happiness, for whole-being, we need to make better use of what the mind and body respectively have to offer us.

Rodin's *The Thinker*

The beautiful bronze sculpture by Auguste Rodin has much to teach us about the mind-body connection. It was a commissioned work, created over the course of many years in the late nineteenth and early twentieth centuries. Initially, its subject was going to be the poet and philosopher Dante and his *Divine Comedy*. Rodin considered depicting the figure clothed, with a long robe, but ultimately decided that he did not want to sculpt a thinker in the image of the typical academic. Instead, he created a thinker with a powerful physical presence. The sculpture is of a muscular nude, crouching with his chin in his hand. In this position it's almost as if he's about to explode like a coil. He's on the verge of taking action. Why did Rodin create a thinker in this pose? Here's what he wrote: "What makes my *Thinker* think is that he thinks not only with his brain, with his knitted brow, his distended nostrils and compressed lips, but with every muscle of his arms, back, and legs, with his clenched fist and gripping toes."[6] In *The Thinker*, mind and body are united.

The Stress Myth

Stress is how our body responds to a threat, real or perceived. Our brain reacts via what's known as the "flight or fight or freeze" response, by signaling for the release of hormones that pump up our heart rate and sharpen our senses. It gears us up to run away, challenge an aggressor, or protect ourselves. Stress has been a health concern and reached pandemic proportions long before we ever heard of coronavirus—in schools, on college campuses, and in the workplace; in the United States and around the world.[7] Prior to the COVID-19 pandemic, the Chinese government issued a declaration saying that their country needs to take better care of rising stress levels among the population. Shortly after that, Australia came out with a similar declaration.

Even before the pandemic, it seems that we were already in trouble when it comes to stress—and now the situation is far worse. These days, with pressures mounting and visions of worst-case scenarios dancing through our minds, it doesn't take much to send us into a state of high alert. Our brain stays ever vigilant, always on the lookout for danger, because there are more and more reasons to be stressed: maybe we don't feel as safe or confident as we once did; perhaps we're anxious about the future of our community, travel, the economy, our income, our children's education, or our health and the health of our loved ones.

What do we do about all this stress? For the past few decades, psychologists and physiologists have studied stress—whether it's in the workplace, on college campuses, or elsewhere—and the conclusions from their research are somewhat surprising and counterintuitive. Most people believe that stress stands in the way of their health and happiness. But what if I told you that we've been blaming the wrong culprit all along? What if I told you that stress, in and of itself, is not the problem? That, in fact, stress is potentially good for us?[8]

Consider the following analogy: You go to the gym and lift some weights. What are you doing to your muscles when you work out? You're stressing them—the muscle fibers break down. We don't see this as a bad thing because we know that stressing our muscles makes them stronger than they were before. Let's say a few days later you lift those dumbbells again, and then a week later you lift slightly heavier ones. You carefully follow a biweekly regimen, work hard for a year, and in time you grow stronger and healthier—thanks to the stress! Stress is not the problem; instead, it is responsible for triggering your body's antifragile system.

The trouble begins when you overzealously decide it's time to get fit. You lift weights, and a minute later more weights, and then again and again. The following day you push yourself to do more reps and then more the day after. Pretty soon you've taken on too much too fast, and that's when you get injured. You become weaker rather than stronger, depleted rather than energized. Your muscles are broken down, but they haven't had a chance to rebuild themselves. The problem, therefore, is not the stress. The problem, rather, is *lack of recovery*.

Whether in the gym, physiologically, or in the world outside, psychologically, the problem is not the presence of stress but rather the absence of recovery.[9] This distinction is potentially life-changing. Stress has always been a part of life. Humans endured stress fifty years ago and five thousand years ago. In the distant past, it was the stress of facing the big, bad wolf or the upcoming winter. Today stress bombards us from different directions: the pandemic's still raging, the car won't start, the kids are fighting. The quarterly report is due, the client's email reads "urgent," coffee just spilled on the laptop. But we can deal with all that stress—in fact we're very good at dealing with it. Just think of all the small fires that you deftly extinguish each day. But the difference between contemporary life and life thousands of years ago is that humans used to have more time for recovery. Today we're "on" all the time and, with packed family and work schedules, we have less time to recuperate. We ignore the fact that recovery is crucial, and not only for our happiness. The combination of stress and lack of recovery is extremely harmful, physically and psychologically.[10]

One way to deal with the stress pandemic could be to exit the rat race, go off to the Himalayas, and meditate eight hours a day. But what if this is not a viable or desirable option for us? Is there an alternative? Yes, there is. We can learn from ambitious, hardworking, and successful people who are also healthy and happy. They, like everyone else, experience stress. However, there's something they do differently: They punctuate their extremely busy lives with periods of downtime—both brief and extended—and the recovery that they experience helps to energize them.[11] Recovery can take place on multiple levels: micro, mid, and macro.

Micro-Level Recovery

Micro-level recovery, as the name suggests, is about taking time out in short stints. It could be taking a fifteen-minute break every two hours for a cup of coffee, a meditation, or a walk around the block. Or it could be scheduling time to read, blocking an hour for exercise, or listening to your favorite music in between meetings with clients. For the recovery to trigger your antifragile system, it has to be real. Taking a break for lunch while also making calls and answering work emails on your phone—that's not real recovery. That's simply more stress.

One of my colleagues, an expert on stress, led a workshop at a trading firm in New York City a few years ago. He was invited to speak to their office because they were going through a stressful period and experiencing a great deal of burnout in the organization. People were choosing to leave the company right and left, others were getting sick and underperforming. My colleague gave a short talk about how stress is not the problem; the problem is the lack of recovery. At the end of his presentation, participants were convinced and eager to move forward. "Tell us, doctor, what do we do?"

He told the traders, "What I'd like you to do is take a fifteen-minute break every two hours."

The employees laughed. "You're joking, right?"

"No, I'm not. Why?"

"We have to have our eyes on that screen at all times. Do you know what can happen in world markets in fifteen minutes? We have lunch in front of those screens. We can't take a break."

"How about five minutes?" My colleague said to them.

"No!"

"How about thirty seconds?"

To that, they agreed.

"OK," he said, "every two hours, take thirty seconds and during those thirty seconds, I want you to close your eyes and take three deep breaths. Five or six seconds in, and then five or six seconds out. Three breaths. If you want to go wild, indulge in four breaths. But," he added, "I'm asking you to do it *consistently*. Every two hours, *every day*. Not just today and tomorrow because you remember that I was here, but make a ritual out of it."

"You've got a deal," they agreed—and they stood by it.

The traders took three to four deep breaths every two hours, and reported that it made a real difference in their overall experience—their wellbeing, productivity, creativity, and energy. Why? Because those thirty seconds of deep breathing provided the much-needed recovery to complement the stress.

The fight, flight, or freeze response is the stress response. Deep breathing enables what Dr. Herbert Benson from Harvard Medical School calls the relaxation response.[12] Often all it takes is three deep breaths for you to make that shift from stress to recovery. Try it! Breathe slowly, gently, and deeply, allowing your belly to rise as you breathe in and to drop as you breathe out. Interestingly, babies naturally breathe this wholesome way most of the time—when they're asleep or awake. Adults, especially when awake, usually do not. This is both a result and a cause of rising levels of stress. In order to exit this downward spiral—where stress leads to shallow breathing, which in turn leads to more stress—we need to engage in more deep breathing. Professor Andrew Weil, founder and director of the Center for Integrative Medicine at the University of Arizona, says: "If I had to limit my advice on healthier living to just one tip, it would be simply to learn how to breathe correctly."[13]

Fortunately, this tool for increased wellbeing is literally under our very noses, and we can use it at any time, in almost every situation. We can focus on breathing more deeply for three to four breaths on our way to work, while sitting in front of the computer, before an important meeting, or whenever we want a moment of calm. Make a point of taking a thirty-second break every two hours to just breathe deeply during your workday—set an alarm if you need a reminder. Practicing deep breathing regularly throughout the day can make a significant difference in the quality of our lives. And if you can find time for regular fifteen-minute breaks every couple of hours, that's even better. I recommend introducing meditation or yoga into your routine, taking a walk, or more strenuous exercise, if you can squeeze it in.

Harvard professor Philip Stone was my role model and mentor. I was his teaching assistant for six years before he handed over his class on positive psychology to me when he retired. Professor Stone taught me many lessons. One of the most important ones was during an offhand moment that took place in 1999, when we were at the first-ever positive psychology conference, held in Lincoln, Nebraska. It was an amazing experience to hear from researchers whose words I had been reading for so long. On the second day, after we broke for lunch, there was a knock on my door. It was Professor Stone. He said, "Let's go for a walk."

"Walk where?" I asked.

He said, "Just walk."

No reason. No rush. No destination necessary. Those two words, *just walk*, are what recovery is all about.

Mid-Level Recovery

Mid-level recovery is about introducing longer breaks into our life, such as taking a day off from work. Even God needed a day off after creating the world! There's an important message here for us mere mortals. People who take a day off from work are not just happier, they're also more productive and more creative overall.[14] Recovery is a good investment.

Getting a good night's sleep is also an important form of mid-level recovery. There is a lot of research on the importance of sleep for our health and happiness.[15] In an attempt to squeeze more out of each twenty-four-hour period, people today are sleeping less than they need to. But as the saying goes, "You cannot skip sleep, you can only borrow against it."[16]

Adults generally need seven to nine hours of sleep per night. Those who do not sleep enough, controlling for other factors, experience more depression and anxiety.[17] Insufficient sleep also makes us irritable and more likely to snap at others. Adults may be able to suppress their crankiness somewhat but still experience the impact of sleep deprivation just as a baby does. This, needless to say, affects the quality of our relationships—we are much more likely to fight with others, upset others, or get upset by others.

Lack of sleep also causes the immune system to weaken, causing us to become more prone to allergies, asthma, colds, and flus. In the case of long-term deprivation, research has shown a significant increase in the likelihood of certain types of cancer and heart disease. In one study, women who slept an average of five hours a night had a 40 percent higher likelihood of a heart attack or coronary artery disease than women who averaged more than seven hours a night.[18]

Additionally, people who do not get sufficient sleep tend to put on weight. When deprived of sleep, the body sends out signals saying it needs more energy. One signal is insulin. After as few as four nights of mild sleep deprivation (meaning around six hours of sleep a night), insulin levels increase significantly.[19] The body then craves high-fat and high-glucose food—that is, junk food. This may lead to obesity, which in turn increases the likelihood of diabetes and other illnesses.

Lack of sleep affects us not just on the inside: It leads to the telltale dark circles around our eyes and a haggard appearance the next day. Ongoing lack of sleep expedites the aging process; sleep keeps us young. When it comes to sex, sleep matters, too. Fatigue is a significant killer of libido. Lack of sleep lowers testosterone levels, and it can cause sexual dysfunction in both men and women.

Sleep also impacts cognitive functioning.[20] Many students—young and old—believe that they perform better even when they don't sleep as much as recommended, because it means they can study more. The same applies to adults who skimp on sleep so that they can get more work done. This may feel like a good short-term solution, and may even be necessary when there is a looming deadline. But over the long haul, it takes a toll, while adequate sleep pays off big-time. Productivity, efficiency, creativity, and memory all increase significantly when we get enough sleep.

If all that is not enough to convince you to turn in earlier, be aware that fatigue is a major cause of accidents[21]: motor skills suffer, drowsiness creeps in, and people fall asleep at work or at the wheel. In the United States, the National Highway Traffic Safety Administration estimates that drowsy driving may be responsible for up to six thousand fatal crashes each year.

So, sleep affects our cognitive functioning, our physiology, and, no surprise—given the connection between mind and body—our psychological wellbeing. Consistent lack of sleep leads to stress without recovery, which then keeps us up at night, and so on, in an unhealthy downward spiral. Sleep expert Sara Mednick, a professor at UC Riverside, writes: "Many of the people we label 'stressed out' are nothing of the sort. They simply need to go to bed."[22]

There's a catch. I've been reading about sleep a lot over the last few years and have sometimes found that doing so actually made my sleep worse! I saw all this research on how important it is to get a full night's sleep and what happens if you don't sleep, and I would go to bed thinking *I have to fall asleep now!* But what happens when you're thinking *I have to fall asleep?* Of course, you're less likely to fall asleep. So, I've learned to just let go of that thought. If you don't fall asleep, don't worry about it. You're still recovering by lying down in bed and taking a break. If you find yourself with insomnia because you're distracted and thinking about tomorrow's to-do list, try reading a book. Don't go online, because the light from the screen makes falling asleep less likely. Don't read upsetting news reports that will push you further away from sleep. You can also try deep, slow breathing. If all else fails and you don't get enough hours at night, take a nap the next day. It's a lot better than nothing. Moreover, while a ninety-minute nap is ideal, as little as fifteen minutes can go a long way toward rejuvenating your mind and lifting your mood. That's fantastic bang for your buck. And if you wake up feeling groggy because you were in the middle of a sleep cycle, wash your face with cold water or take a few quick steps to get the blood flowing. You'll immediately feel recharged and ready to go.

Macro-Level Recovery

Finally, there is macro-level recovery. Whether it's going camping, taking time off to just read, or doing absolutely nothing for a few days or weeks, your body and mind need longer breaks from the daily grind as a form of re-cuperation. A recent study found that more than half of Americans do not use all their vacation days.[23] Among those who do take vacation, more than 40 percent re-main tethered to the office, by checking work email, for example. Without proper recovery, happiness and perfor-mance levels drop. But people who take time away from work are overall more productive and more creative.[24] It's no coincidence that there is an etymological connec-tion between *recreation* and *creation*. It is when we recreate that we're most poised to create.

Taking time off—real time off—is extremely difficult to do, especially for type A, ambitious individuals. We (and I say *we*, because I'm type A, too), feel that if we take a break we're going to miss out on an opportunity.

We'll be out of the loop. Other people are working hard and continuing to get ahead, and we're not. To change your perspective, try thinking about it in the context of an elite Formula 1 driver. A race car zooms around the track again and again—but it can't complete a race without making pit stops. If a driver were to say, *Uh-oh, if I stop now, the other drivers will take over. I'm not going to take a pit stop*, what would happen? Inevitably, a dangerous situation—either the tires would blow out or the car would run out of fuel. This is the equivalent of burnout. In your personal life and professional life, succumbing to FOMO—the fear of missing out—leads to COBO: the certainty of burning out.

Whether it's on the micro-level, mid-level, or macro-level, if we don't take those recovery pit stops, we will inevitably burn out or spin out—and then it becomes even more difficult to get back on track. Even the most well-tuned race car can't go full speed ahead indefinitely. No matter how strong and resilient you are, you still need those breaks. Moreover, it's during those breaks that you become stronger. And this is how stress can have an upside: Recovery activates our antifragile system— helping us become better, healthier, and happier. Exactly how often you need recovery breaks, and for how long, is more a question for me-search rather than research. Now, the research indicates that on average, we need to pause for recovery every ninety minutes or so, take at least one day off a week, and spend a couple of weeks vacationing a year,[25] but you can experiment with how much you personally need. Give yourself a break!

Single-Tasking

Single-tasking, as the name suggests, is dedicating yourself to doing just one thing at any given time. It's about ignoring the siren song of the many other must-dos that beckon you all the time. To lower your stress, you'll want to reduce multitasking and, whenever possible, engage in single-tasking. *Tal,* you may be thinking, *I multitask so I can get more done. If I can get more items crossed off my list, I'll be less stressed out.* While progress and productivity can certainly contribute to your overall happiness, and while some multitasking is necessary and unavoidable, too much multitasking can increase stress and deplete your energy. So even if you do multitask, introducing single-tasking breaks during the day—staying fully engaged in one activity at a time—can help a great deal. Single-tasking relaxes your body, focuses your mind, and gives you the strength to continue.

It doesn't matter what these single-tasking activities are—it could be spending time with a family member, friend, or colleague and giving them your full attention, or answering emails and nothing else, or dancing and being fully immersed in the music. I call these single-tasking experiences "islands of sanity" because they provide some sane recovery periods in our crazy-busy, multitasking, multilayered world.

Exercise

A great deal of research points to one simple conclusion: It's very important to be physically active.[26] Although on some level we all know this, exercise is typically one of the first things that people let slide when they're busy and stressed.

I ask my college students when they are least likely to exercise and why. Almost unanimously, they say during exam period. They figure that they need the time to study and cannot afford to spend time exercising. My response is that times of stress are when exercise is most crucial. Exercise is among the most powerful forms of recovery from psychological stress, because it is extremely effective for dealing with anxiety.

Regular exercise—as little as thirty minutes of aerobic exercise three times a week—has the same effect on individuals with major depression as our most powerful psychiatric medication.[27] Exercise is equally helpful for individuals with dysthymia, a lower grade, longer lasting kind of depression. In fact, exercise works in the same way as medication, releasing norepinephrine, serotonin, and dopamine, the feel-good chemicals in our brain.[28]

When I saw these and other results on the impact of physical activity, I initially thought to myself that exercising is like taking an antidepressant. But as I continued to think about it I realized that's not exactly the case. It's not that exercising is like taking an antidepressant, but rather that *not exercising is like taking a depressant*. This is more than a semantic difference. We were not made, born, created, evolved to be sedentary creatures. We aren't supposed to sit at home all day in front of a computer, with no physical activity. We were built to move, literally born to run—whether to run after an antelope for lunch, or away from a lion so that we don't become lunch. Today it's all too easy to barely move our muscles for stretches of time, and swiping our finger across a screen doesn't exactly count. When we frustrate a need, whether it's the need for oxygen, vitamins, sleep, or exercise, we pay a high price. And because mind and body are one, the physical frustration leads to psychological frustration.

We all have a base level of wellbeing, determined by our genes and early experiences—both of which are out of our control. If we don't exercise, we lower that base level, compromising our God-given or genetically-given hand, which is why not exercising is like taking a depressant.

Given the impact of physical exercise, does it mean that we don't need antidepressants, that we can throw the pills out of our medicine cabinets? Not at all. Exercise is not a cure-all, and sometimes medication is the best route to take. At the same time, the research strongly suggests that we need to start looking at physical activity as a very effective psychological intervention.[29]

Sixteenth-century philosopher Francis Bacon, the father of modern science, wrote, "Nature, to be commanded, must be obeyed." Our nature is such that we need regular exercise. It's always important, but especially during challenging times.

Move It Move It

Exercise doesn't just mean an intense sweat session at the gym. More generally, movement is essential for our wellbeing. Research out of the University of Cambridge in England shows that people who move more often tend to be happier. This is true even if they have a desk job, but every twenty to thirty minutes they just get up and walk around—a micro recovery. More and more doctors are suggesting that "sitting is the new smoking," and while this may be exaggerating a little bit, it's not by much. Sitting for long periods of time is unhealthy.[30] As a rule of thumb, don't sit for longer than thirty minutes without getting up and moving. Climb a flight of stairs, walk up and down the halls, go to the bathroom—but move. Movement is critical for physical and mental health.

Are you exercising regularly? If you haven't been, don't feel guilty about it. Just go out and do it! Remember, movement is in your nature. It's difficult enough to increase our wellbeing. Don't make happiness harder for yourself by struggling against nature.

Now, what does regular exercise mean? Recommendations vary, with the minimum being thirty minutes of aerobic exercise three times a week and the optimal being forty-five minutes five times a week. If you do high-intensity interval training (HIIT), you can derive similar physical and psychological benefits in shorter sessions. There are thousands of HIIT programs that you can find online. Adding some strength training to the mix is important, especially as we grow older. My exercise regime is usually three weekly sessions of HIIT with irregular weight training scattered here and there; however, in difficult times—such as now—I add a weekly aerobic session and two muscle-strengthening activities to the mix. I intentionally move more often because I feel like I need it.

Your exercise regime could involve brisk walking—even if it's just walking around your apartment. It could include jumping on a trampoline, which is what I like to do. Mini-trampolines don't take up much space, are relatively inexpensive, and are easy to find online. If you have a treadmill at home, dust it off and lace up your sneakers, or just go for a run outside, go swimming, or play basketball. Find high-intensity circuit training (HICT) sessions online that combine cardio with muscle-strengthening exercises. Whatever you decide to do, pencil in a few blocks of time on your calendar, so that you can move it move it.

Dance

Dance is actually the most powerful exercise for increasing happiness! It's very difficult to dance and be somber; we usually can't help but smile when we shake our bodies to the beat of our favorite music. And given the facial feedback hypothesis, that smile is internalized and we become happier. Our posture when we dance also impacts our mood. Have a dance party at home with your kids or friends, take a virtual ballroom lesson with your partner, or take a dance class or do Zumba on your own. Whatever is your favorite way to boogie, go and get your exercise fix. It works like a drug without the side effects, or rather with plenty of positive side effects.

Children and Exercise

Exercising has positive effects for people of all ages. Research by John Ratey, a Harvard Medical School psychiatrist, shows that in schools that introduce regular exercise, kids are happier. They are also less violent: Physical and verbal aggression goes down by more than 60 percent just by incorporating exercise into the day. Children that exercise do better academically and become more productive, creative, and engaged. Exercise on its own, or as an adjunct treatment, can help with attention deficit hyperactivity disorder (ADHD).[31] Whether your kids spend their mornings in school or at home, I urge you to make exercise a mandatory part of their day.

Bruegel's "Children's Games"

Flemish artist Pieter Bruegel, one of the great Renaissance artists of the sixteenth century, created a beautiful oil painting called *Children's Games*. It depicts what life used to look like in the Belgian villages: children playing outside, running around, doing handstands and somersaults, and riding piggyback. This whole painting is a celebration of movement. It reminds me of my childhood in Israel, where I grew up spending countless hours playing outside. Like many Mediterranean countries, Israel has siesta time, between two and four PM, but as soon as the clock struck four, we would run outside and play hide-and-seek, soccer, or tag. We moved and played constantly until dinnertime. Today, kids' lives are very different, with much more finger movement perhaps, but far less whole-body activities.

How can we learn from this painting and apply more movement to our lives? Now is as good a time as any for us to encourage our children to move, and for us as adults to capture the free spirit of childhood and start new rituals around exercise and play. For me, this painting is an inspiration to move a lot more, and move with joy.

Aging

The impact of physical exercise on aging is undeniable. A meta-analysis on the relationship between physical activity and aging shows that regular exercise reduces the likelihood of Alzheimer's and dementia by 52 percent.[32] This is the case even if you start a workout regimen later in life. There is no medication that even comes close to having such an effect. When I heard of this study, I immediately called my mother. I said, "Mom, you know how until now I recommended that you exercise? Well, I'm no longer recommending it. I'm *demanding* it." Normally, I would never talk to my mom like that. However, I did then. Why? Because her mother, my grandmother, died with Alzheimer's disease. My mom's aunt, my grandmother's sister, also died with Alzheimer's. Unfortunately, there is a hereditary component to the illness. So, I told my mom, "You have to exercise. If not for yourself, then for your children and grandchildren." I'm relieved that she took the advice to heart and started to exercise religiously, continuing to do so even during the COVID lockdown.

If you're not already exercising, then regardless of your age, start moving. Do it gradually—it's better to err on the side of starting too slow rather than too fast—ideally, with the guide of a coach or a doctor. If possible, take up activities that you enjoy because you are naturally more likely to persist with those. Exercise is always vital, and especially so during times when stress tends to be higher.

Blue Zones

Dan Buettner from *National Geographic*, alongside other researchers, studied the Blue Zones—areas in the world where people live the longest.[33] These include Ikaria, a small island in Greece; Okinawa, Japan; Loma Linda, California; the Mediterranean island Sardinia, Italy; and Nicoya, Costa Rica. These places have five to seven times more centenarians—people above age one hundred—than anywhere else. Buettner wrote *The Blue Zones* with the purpose of introducing the world's best practices in health and longevity, so that we can apply them in our lives. In his book, he concludes that "if we adopted the right lifestyle, we could add at least ten good years and suffer a fraction of the diseases that kill us prematurely." Many of the ideas that Buettner identifies are relevant not just for physical wellbeing, but also for psychological wellbeing—for happiness.

It probably won't come as a surprise that people in the Blue Zones habitually engage in exercise. Yet they don't go to the gym; most don't have gyms anywhere nearby. Instead, they exercise through the course of their normal activities. Sometimes they walk up a mountain. Sometimes they just walk a long way to see a friend or go to a store. By necessity, they lift and haul heavy loads. In our modern world, we have it too easy. A remote control is always available, food is always a phone call away. And lifting our hand, even if it's to carry a whole smartphone, is not enough exercise.

It's interesting that there isn't a universal diet among residents of the Blue Zones, but there are universal principles: eating natural whole foods rather than processed foods, for example, as well as consuming an abundance of fruits, vegetables, and nuts. Moreover, it turns out that it's not just the quality of food that matters, but also quantity. Blue Zones residents eat in moderation. For instance, in Okinawa they have a saying that they utter before each meal: "Eat until you're 80 percent full." In contrast, most of us often eat until we're full—and then some.

We can find the other SPIRE elements in the lives of the Blue Zones residents. For example, they enjoy a sense of meaning in life (spiritual wellbeing) as well as deep friendships and family connections (relational wellbeing). At the same time, Buettner emphasizes that we don't need to do it all, nor do we need to introduce radical action into our lives to gain significant benefits. We can focus on any of the elements of SPIRE, and then within that element—say physical wellbeing—small changes can make a big difference. For example, cutting down slightly on the quantity we eat, or adding extra vegetables or nuts to our diet can go a long way. And when it comes to exercising, Buettner talks about the value of *inconveniencing* ourselves in small ways, by getting up rather than using the remote, taking the stairs rather than the elevator, walking once in a while rather than driving everywhere.

Consistency Is the Key

There may be mornings when you wake up and feel like you have zero energy. We've all been there. One of my students said to me, "There are days when I'm capable of doing everything that I want—exercise, yoga, meditation—but then there are days when I really feel like doing nothing." My student is not alone in feeling this way. The roller coaster is real, even more so during stressful periods—one day you may have an abundance of energy, and the next day a shortage. Certainly, I have days when I just want to hide in my room and do nothing. One of the challenges of feeling down is averting the downward spiral—we're feeling low, so we say to ourselves, *Why bother?*; we stop exercising and prioritizing recoveries, and as a result, we feel even worse, and so on.

The downward spiral often manifests in procrastination, pushing off things that don't absolutely need to be done now until later . . . and later. So, what does the research recommend on procrastination?[34] Try a strategy called the five-minute takeoff by saying to yourself: *Even though I don't feel like doing this now, I'm gonna do it anyway for just five minutes*. For example, walk or dance or play ball for five minutes, and you'll discover that more often than not, these five minutes will lead to five more, and so on. The five-minute takeoff applies to more than exercising. For example, on days when I don't feel like writing, I often turn to the five-minute takeoff. Soon after I start, within a few minutes, I get into a rhythm and can then write for two hours or more. I find the energy comes once I'm actually in the process.

The mistake that many procrastinators make is believing that motivation precedes action. In other words, they believe that in order to do something, you first have to feel inspired. That's not the case. Those who don't procrastinate, or procrastinate less, have the opposite model. They realize that it's not about inspiration first; rather, it's about action preceding motivation. Just by starting, just by doing, you're more likely to reach a state of mind where you're excited and propelled to keep going, even if you were feeling down. Sometimes we need to fake it until we make it, or as social psychologist Amy Cuddy says, "Fake it until we become it."[35]

Exercising three times per week on a regular basis, even if you miss a session occasionally, will make a difference. Earlier we talked about how a recovery break of as little as thirty seconds during the day makes a difference. It really does, if you do it regularly. That's the key: Small changes make a big difference *if applied consistently.* If I had the option, say, of going on a one-time weekend-long meditation retreat versus meditating for five minutes daily on an ongoing basis, I'd opt for the latter; if the option was between running fifteen miles once a week or five miles three times a week, I'd go for

the shorter runs. Why? Because change applied consistently is what boosts happiness long-term, much more
so than occasional spikes of activity.

THE SPIRE CHECK-IN

Physical Wellbeing

Go through the three steps of the SPIRE Check-In–ascribe, describe, and prescribe–focusing on physical wellbeing. Begin by reflecting on the following questions:

How physically active are you?

Do you take care of your body?

Do you take time for rest and recovery?

How do you deal with stress?

Based on your reflections, determine the degree to which you experience physical wellbeing and then *ascribe* a score from 1 to 10, with 1 being very little or very infrequently, and 10 being very much or very often. After ascribing a score, in writing *describe* why you gave yourself that score. Then, *prescribe* a way to increase your score by just one point at first. Examples may include three exercise sessions a week, thirty seconds of deep breathing every two hours, single-tasking at least one hour each day, taking the batteries out of the remote control, and more. Keep checking in with yourself once a week.

Chapter 3

—

Intellectual Wellbeing

*The greatest mistake you can make in life is
continually fearing that you'll make one.*

—Elbert Hubbard

W hen Aristotle, the wise Greek philosopher, described a human being as a rational animal, he suggested that our ability to think and to reason—our intellect—defines us. But is this defining quality, which Aristotle argues distinguishes us as a species, good for our happiness? There is a common belief that to be happy we should strive for the mindset of a grazing cow—that without thinking we will be free from worrying, and we can just be . . . happy. After all, the argument goes, thinking often takes us down the spiral of brooding and gloom. However, for most if not all people, just living as an animal—gratifying physical needs and little else—would lead to much unhappiness in the long-term. How, then, do we best use our intellectual capacities so that they contribute to, rather than detract from, our happiness?

Intellectual wellbeing has several facets, and in this chapter I will discuss three of them. First, intellectual wellbeing is about fostering your innate invincible curiosity, your natural desire to learn more. Second, it's about the value of delving into subjects deeply, both as a source of pleasure and to sharpen your thinking. Third, it's about being open to making more mistakes. Paradoxically, it's when we learn to embrace failure—recognizing it as a vital experience rather than something to fear or reject—that we prime ourselves to reach new heights.

Cultivating Curiosity

We are born innately curious about the world around us and within us, but as we get older this instinct is sometimes stifled—often by well-meaning educators, be they parents or teachers. Psychologist Mihaly Csikszentmihalyi writes:

> Neither parents nor schools are very effective at teaching the young to find pleasure in the right things. Adults, themselves often deluded by infatuation with fatuous models, conspire in the deception. They make serious tasks seem dull and hard, and frivolous ones exciting and easy. Schools generally fail to teach how exciting, how mesmerizingly beautiful science or mathematics can be; they teach the routine of literature or history rather than the adventure.[1]

The focus on extrinsic measures of success such as grades and trophies, standardized tests and competition, is taking its toll on our intrinsic passion for and love of learning. The enthusiasm and excitement children display in asking questions and learning often give way to dullness and boredom around schoolwork. Needless to say, there is a lack of intellectual wellbeing in this way of learning. In the words of educator Neil Postman,

"Children enter school as question marks and leave school as periods." This approach to learning—and often to life as a whole—remains as these children grow up and find little engagement at work or home. We fail to make the most of life, and tragically pass on this unexcited and uninspired approach to learning to the next generation.

Fortunately, it's very hard to annihilate curiosity altogether. Rather, it is put to sleep, lying dormant—eagerly awaiting the moment it will be woken. The burning desire to learn may at times be reduced to a tiny spark that, in its diminished state, isn't powerful enough to make us passionate about life—and yet the spark still possesses the potential to ignite a fire. Albert Einstein, whose passion for learning was one of his defining characteristics, wrote: "It is, in fact, nothing short of a miracle that the modern methods of instruction have not yet entirely strangled the holy curiosity of inquiry." We should not take this miracle for granted, however; we should not just continue with business as usual. Instead, we ought to do our best to rekindle the remaining sparks of curiosity, to reignite our passion for learning.

How do we return to our natural state of curiosity if we've left it behind? Perhaps the most formidable barrier standing in the way of a return to curiosity is the false belief that some of us are simply not curious—that for some people the desire to ask questions, to learn, and to grow has been extinguished, or was never there in the first place. The problem with this mistaken belief is that it becomes a self-fulfilling prophecy, thwarting any attempt to discover an interest or a passion. Without seeking there can be no finding.

The first step to reignite the love of learning involves faith—faith in the existence of an innate and invincible curiosity. To categorically state "I don't like learning" is analogous to declaring "I don't like eating." We might not like sardines or cucumbers, but we are so constituted that we derive pleasure from eating, at least some things. Similarly, we might not like studying calculus or ancient languages, but our nature dictates that we are capable of deriving pleasure from learning. Asking questions and discovering new things satisfy our inquisitive nature just as food and water satisfy our physical nature. Just as food is necessary to survive and thrive, and so we desire it, so, too, is learning and growing, and so we naturally crave it. As babies, if we were devoid of curiosity we would not venture out of our crib—we would not learn how to crawl or walk, grab or embrace.[2]

If you are intent on rekindling your love of learning, the question you should be asking is not *whether* you like to learn, but rather *what and how* you like to learn. You may be inclined to explore the world of numbers and symbols, whereas someone else may be drawn to art and music; your interest may be piqued by humanity's origins and evolution, or you may be kept up at night by questions about the meaning and purpose of it all; there are those fascinated by human psychology and others by animal physiology. Fortunately, our world is so rich and multifaceted that there is no shortage of possibilities to engage and study.

In addition to removing the false belief that your curiosity may have been completely extinguished, another step that can help in reigniting the passion for learning is to fake it until you make it. Cornell psychologist Daryl Bem conducted research demonstrating how we form attitudes about ourselves in the same way that we form attitudes about others—namely, through observation.[3] If we see a man helping others, we conclude that he is kind; if we see a woman standing up for her beliefs, we conclude that she is principled and courageous. Similarly, we draw conclusions about ourselves by observing our own behavior. When we act kindly or courageously, our attitudes are likely to shift in the direction of our action, and we tend to feel, and see ourselves as, kinder and more courageous. Through this mechanism, which Bem calls Self-Perception Theory, behaviors can change attitudes over time. And since curiosity is an attitude toward life, we can change it through our behaviors: By observing our own curiosity, we can actually become more curious.

So, if you have lost this loving feeling toward learning, fake it until you make it. Ask friends or colleagues questions in the areas of their expertise, read articles or watch lectures about a topic of which you have little knowledge, and go deeper into a topic that you are already familiar with. Since the spark of curiosity is already there, it won't be long before the passion for learning is reignited.

We can acquire a taste for knowledge. An analogy: There is a great deal of research showing how babies and adults acquire tastes for particular foods.[4] For example, a two-year-old might initially reject and not like cucumbers, but after trying them a dozen times or so she will begin to acquire a taste for cucumbers. A middle-aged man who was never exposed to cucumbers may not initially like the taste, but after tasting it a few dozen times—his brain is less flexible than that of the toddler—he will in all likelihood begin to enjoy cucumbers. It is through trials that we stretch our palate, diversifying the range of our desired tastes and textures. In the same way, we can learn to be more curious and open to experiences—to expand and diversify the range of our exploration—by trying new ideas and experiences. Just as our taste buds metaphorically expand, so do our minds. Ralph Waldo Emerson wrote that "The mind, once stretched by a new idea, never returns to its original dimensions." Begin stretching. The benefits are manifold. By consistently stretching your mind, you are essentially making yourself more antifragile, better able to learn from and overcome difficulties. And given the mind-body connection we discussed in the previous chapter, it is not just your mind that will benefit from being more curious, your body will, too.

Lillian Smith, the twentieth-century American author who bravely fought against segregation and for gender and racial equality, wrote: "When you stop learning, stop listening, stop looking and asking questions, always new questions, then it is time to die." Smith advocated for ongoing curiosity, lifelong learning. But isn't her verdict of a death sentence for the end of curiosity a bit harsh? Yes, it probably is. And being a fiction writer, she sought, and found, the dramatic. However, there is some truth in the drama. For instance, health researchers Gary Swan and Dorit Carmelli demonstrated the relationship between curiosity and longevity.[5] In their study, controlling for other factors, aging adults who were curious were likely to live longer than those who were not. Curiosity may kill the cat, but it seems to prolong life for humans.

Ask Yourself Questions

We can also point the lens of curiosity at ourselves. The ancient Greek philosopher Socrates, considered the father of the Western intellectual tradition, led his students toward insight and understanding not by lecturing and providing answers, but by exploring and asking questions. This pedagogical approach is what we've come to call the Socratic method. Thousands of miles from where Socrates lived and more than a hundred years earlier, Confucius, considered the father of the Eastern intellectual tradition, situated inquiry at the center of his philosophy as well. A famous Chinese proverb that is attributed to Confucius, or at the very least is inspired by him, says the following: "He who asks a question is a fool for five minutes; he who does not ask a question remains a fool forever."

Asking questions is something we naturally do, and that's a good thing because it helps us learn and grow. Less helpful, especially when facing difficulties and hardships, is our tendency to focus our questions on what isn't working—to inquire about the empty rather than full part of the glass. For example, if I am going through a difficult time, the questions I am likely to ask—or be asked—are "What is not going well in your life?" or "Why are you anxious?" If my partner and I are struggling in our relationship, we (and those who seek to help us) might ask, "What is not working in the relationship?" or "What's behind all the quarreling?" If a company isn't meeting its goals, the questions that management or external consultants usually ask are "What are the organization's weaknesses?" or "What are the barriers that stand in its way?"

These are valid, important questions, but mounting evidence suggests that focusing on the problems is not enough and that if we want to fulfill our potential, whether personally, interpersonally, or organizationally, we need to go beyond what's lacking and also examine the full part of the glass. David Cooperrider, cofounder of the field of appreciative inquiry, notes that "We live in a world that our questions create." If we are to create the best possible world for ourselves and others we need to ask positive questions: "We find that the more positive the question we ask, the more long-lasting and successful the change effort."[6]

To increase the likelihood of positive change, instead of focusing on the things that aren't working, you can flip the focus of your questions. Even as you go through difficult times, you can ask yourself: What *is* going well in my life? What are some potential sources of calm? What *is* working in my relationship and where do we thrive together? What are the organization's strengths and what is its competitive advantage?

After highlighting the things that are working—whether in your life, your relationship, or your organization— you can proceed to ask: What can I learn and apply from the things that are going well and that are working?

A question is like a flashlight that illuminates and draws your attention to a defined area. Beyond the circle of light, everything else exists in darkness. If you ask too limited a question, even if you spend much time and effort answering it, you may not find what you're looking for. Making decisions requires that you reflect on the possibilities in front of you—but you can't reflect on what you can't yet see. The fundamental way to expand your options is in your choice of questions.

12 New Questions

Here is a list of questions that have been helpful to me and to others. You can use these to help guide you through a difficult situation or toward a goal. Keep in mind that the list is far from exhaustive, and there are many additional questions that may be better suited for different people and for different situations. Just as you spend a lot of time and effort honing your answering skills, practice doing the same with your inquiry skills. As you experiment and become better at asking—testing different questions, trying and trying again—new paths will open up to you. These are just a few questions that can foster your curiosity, broaden your vision, and in turn contribute to your whole person wellbeing.

1. When am I at my happiest?
2. How can I become happier?
3. Where do I experience meaning in my life?
4. How can I find more meaning?
5. What positive habits do I have?
6. How can I introduce more positive habits into my life?
7. What do I love to learn?
8. How can I further indulge my curiosity?
9. What is working in my relationships?
10. What can I do to make my relationships better?
11. When do I feel most joy?
12. How can I bring more joy to my life?

Deep Learning

When I started college, the first course I took my freshman year was speed-reading. It was offered to incoming students the week before the actual school year began in anticipation of a heavy workload. It was an excellent course, and thanks to it I was able to get through hundreds of pages a week, which I wouldn't have been able to do otherwise. That course kept me in good stead throughout my college- and graduate-school career, and even today, it helps me keep up with the daily NBA news and the ever-changing political landscape. However, there's an even more important course Harvard should have offered, one that I think all universities and workplaces should offer: slow-reading. In other words, not a class in superficial learning, but in deep learning.

I did eventually learn to slow-read from my adviser, the philosopher Robert Nozick. Every week, he would assign a short excerpt to read and ask me to write about it. Then, for one hour, he would choose one paragraph of my response and, alongside the assigned excerpt that I read, dissect it to bits and pieces. I was able to see how many layers of meaning were wrapped up in every sentence. The impact of this exercise was remarkable. I learned to read slowly and think deeply.

What, though, are the benefits of deeply engaging with a text, or, for that matter, with a work of art or with nature? Why should you spend time reading a paragraph over and over again, contemplating a beautiful painting, or reflecting on the tree outside your window? Aren't you wasting your time? Given that there is so much great material out there, shouldn't you get through as much as possible in the short time that you have? Well, if your primary concern is getting through as much as you can and checking all the boxes, then foregoing depth for breadth is the way to go. However, if your primary concern is cultivating happiness, wholebeing, then you ought to spend at least some of the time that you have digging deep.

First and foremost, deep learning can provide you with a great deal of joy and pleasure. When I was in high school, we had to read *Crime and Punishment*. I read it, but I didn't enjoy it. Moreover, I read the Cliff's Notes (don't tell my English teacher), the shorter version that explains what you most need to know in order to do well on an exam. But today, having returned to Dostoevsky without deadlines, I enjoy this work a great deal more. When I read, I get to luxuriate in the pleasure of engaging with the brilliant mind of Dostoevsky, visiting nineteenth-century St. Petersburg, while contemplating the nature of our moral sense. There's no need for speed—and there's plenty of time to learn, grow, savor, and appreciate. I am reminded of Henry David Thoreau's words, written around the same time as *Crime and Punishment*: "Life is too short to be in a hurry."

A second benefit of deep learning is that it can help you become more successful in other areas of your life. My European ancestors were successful businessmen. They didn't go to business school; in fact, they didn't go to college, and most of them didn't even attend high school. When I was growing up, I asked my grandfather their secret. He told me that though they didn't receive much formal education, nonetheless they were scholars.

My ancestors intensively studied the Hebrew Bible and the Talmud daily, whether on their own, with a Rabbi, a family member, or a friend. They would analyze a single passage for hours on end and engage in lively disagreements about their translation of the original text from Hebrew or Aramaic. Sometimes they would spend days talking about the intention of a sentence, or about the true meaning of a single word.

Deep learning made these scholars not just theologically smart, but also street smart. The two worlds—the material and the spiritual—seem so far apart, but they're not. The ability to study and know a biblical text translates quite readily into the ability to understand a business model, review a contract, or evaluate a potential client. Moreover, the energy—the positive, joyful energy—is almost always evident in a place of deep learning. By fully exercising our intellectual capacities we become both smarter and happier.

Just as deep learning can help us professionally, it can also have a positive effect on our relationships. Believe it or not, our ability to know a text and appreciate its complexities can deepen our relationships with a romantic partner, a friend, a colleague, or a child. How, though, does the way we read impact the way we interact with others? We have one brain, one neural system, that functions within these multiple domains. The more we reinforce the neural connections for superficial learning in one area, the more we rely on them in other areas of our life. The average amount of time that people spend on a webpage today is seven seconds. We get a glimpse of it, glean what we can, and then click to the next. It leads us to the ongoing need for new stimulation and novelty. This translates to a short attention span, boredom, and a constant need for novelty in other areas of life, like relationships. In other words, an inability to deeply engage with a text beyond the superficial translates into an inability to truly know a person—leading to skin-deep relationships and inevitable boredom. In contrast, when we take the time to read at length and reengage with rich material, we constantly find more nuances and distinctions, and understand at an increasingly deeper level. Once we train these "muscles," we can also apply them to interpersonal relationships and become much more adept at engaging deeply with people.

There is no text that is as multifaceted, rich, and potentially interesting as another person. A person is quite literally a whole world unto him or herself. You'll find that there's always something new to learn about a person. However, we need to practice. Knowing what we do about the way our brain works, I think it's fair to say that the high levels of disengagement in relationships we see throughout society today are at least partially a result of our reluctance to exercise those deep-learning muscles.

The fact that we have quick access to so much content today—on our small smartphones, we have a fire hose of articles, posts, podcasts, webinars, courses, songs, movies, and books always at our fingertips—doesn't help deep learning. The French philosopher Voltaire wrote, "The multitude of books is making us ignorant." Note that he was living in the eighteenth century. Information today is being generated and disseminated at a breathtaking pace. In 2010, Eric Schmidt, who was then CEO of Google, said that *every two days* humans create more information than was created from the dawn of civilization to 2003. People receive more information daily than they were exposed to in a lifetime back when Voltaire was writing. And yet Voltaire's words were prescient. He was speaking to the phenomenon that when there are so many choices, so many distractions, we do not focus, concentrate, go deep, and really learn.

When there are so many options, it can be hard to decide what to focus on. Here the old adage is true: Quality is more important than quantity. If you find that you get sucked into internet surfing, set limits: restrict yourself to a certain amount of time or certain number of articles, and that's it. If you can't listen to every podcast on your list, it's OK to just stick with one. The key is to be selective and not get caught up in the fear of missing out. Less is more when it comes to learning.

The Beginner's Mind

To develop intellectual wellbeing, I urge you to put down your phone (stop doomscrolling!) and pick up a book. In fact, I urge you to commit long-term to an ambitious book. English Professor Marjorie Garber is an expert on Shakespeare and has been reading and teaching Shakespeare for decades. And yet, she says that every time she reads Shakespeare, she discovers something she hadn't fully comprehended or internalized before. This is what great literature has to offer us. Here is my project for you: Pick up that great book you've always wanted to tackle—it may already be on your bookshelf—and read it. Then re-read it. Study it again at an even deeper level. Personally,

I can't count how many times I've read Lao Tzu's *Tao Te Ching*, Mary Ann Evans's *Middlemarch*, and Aristotle's *Nicomachean Ethics*. Each time I read one of these books, the effect on my life is profound; I better understand—and more deeply appreciate—the book, the world, and myself. Especially when going through rough times, these timeless books provide me with a stabilizing anchor.

Curiosity and deep learning go hand in hand, as they nurture our intellectual wellbeing, and by extension our wholebeing. As you engage and reengage with your book, try to come to it as if for the first time—this mindset is known as "beginner's mind." It's a form of active mindfulness often associated with meditation. The fundamental characteristic of beginner's mind is curiosity. Zen master Shunryu Suzuki writes: "In the beginner's mind there are many possibilities, but in the expert's there are few."[7]

Psychologist Ellen Langer, one of my mentors, for years has studied ways to enter this state of curiosity. She urges us to "draw novel distinctions"—to notice new things we hadn't before and observe details we previously might not have paid attention to when considering an object that is seemingly familiar.[8] Langer's research shows that cultivating this state boosts happiness and health, promotes self-esteem and motivation, and improves memory, learning, and creativity. It is this state of intellectual openness and flexibility that best prepares us to overcome barriers and grow from hardship.

To be sure, learning can go beyond reading. It can include engaging with the beauty of nature: going out for a walk and really observing what's out there. It can include learning to move your body in ways that are challenging for you. During the COVID lockdown, I spent time practicing more dance moves. Trust me, it's nothing you want to see, but the fact that I had to learn, that my cognitive muscles were engaged (in addition to my physical muscles) yielded much benefit, contributing to my intellectual wellbeing (and to my kids' wholebeing, as they laughed watching me dance—laughed at me rather than with me, I suspect). Whatever medium you choose to study—a book, a work of art, a dance, the natural world, or anything else—the most important element of intellectual wellbeing is nurturing your ability to engage in a deep way.

Learn to Fail or Fail to Learn

As you cultivate your intellectual wellbeing—as you curiously engage with life's treasures—there are two more things that I hope will happen to you. First, that you fail more. I genuinely don't think you fail enough. Second, that you embrace failure. Very few of us appreciate the importance of failure for success and happiness.

Imagine parents who love their baby so intensely that they don't want their child to ever get hurt in the slightest, so they decide they won't ever let her fall down. Every time the baby is about to stand up and take a step, they pick her up immediately. After all, they know that she'll fall, possibly hurt herself, and probably cry. The cost of shielding the child from falling? The child would never learn how to walk.

Young children are not afraid of failure; for them it is a natural part of living—that is why they get right up again after a spill, why they scribble joyfully on the way to learning to write their name, and why they create a huge mess on the floor (and their face) before they learn to eat with utensils. And yet, as we get older and become more self-conscious, instead of focusing our energy on trying and trying again, we concentrate on avoiding failure and preserving an image of perfection.

Failure is essential for learning and growing. Psychologist Dean Simonton of UC Davis researched many of the greatest artists and scientists in history, including Mozart, Shakespeare, Albert Einstein, and Marie Curie. He found that the one element common to all these visionaries is that they failed more times than most people.[9]

Thomas Edison, one of the most creative and productive inventors of all time, patented a whopping 1,093 inventions, including the light bulb, a sound recording system, and the battery. When Edison was working on his battery, generating power from a cell, a journalist came to interview him and asked him about his progress. The journalist remarked that Edison had been working on this project for a long time and suggested that he turn his attention to other inventions since he had already failed ten thousand times. Edison responded: "I have not failed. I've just found ten thousand ways that won't work."

One of Edison's most famous sayings is, "I failed my way to success." So, yes, Thomas Edison certainly deserves a place in the Hall of Fame of luminaries. He also deserves an honorary place in the Hall of Fame of failures. It's no coincidence that the people who achieve the most also fail the most.

Babe Ruth is familiar to most Americans as one of the greatest baseball players of all time. For decades he held the record for most home runs: 714 in his career. Although he was an incredible batter, a lesser-known fact is that for five years Ruth was at the top of the league in strikeouts. In other words, just like Edison, he was exceptional for both hits and misses.

What does this mean for us? There is much research on the importance of optimism, of saying yes to achieve success. Saying yes to new ideas, yes to possibilities, and yes to opportunities is the foundation of thriving. But to build on that foundation, another word similar to *yes* is critical— and that is the word *yet*.[10] Yes, I believe I can invent a new battery. I have conducted thousands of experiments and haven't come up with a solution . . . yet. Yes, I can create a thriving business. It is not making money . . . yet. Yes, I want to make a difference through politics. I have not been elected to office . . . yet. *Yes* is the word that starts us off; *yet* is the word that keeps us going . . . and going, and going. And while success is never guaranteed, *yet* is the word that takes us from breaking down to building up, from fragility to antifragility.

In the words of Theodore Roosevelt,

> It is not the critic who counts: not the man who points out how the strong man stumbles or where the doer of deeds could have done them better. The credit belongs to the man who is actually in the arena . . . who errs, who comes short again and again, because there is no effort without error and shortcoming . . . who, at the best, knows, in the end, the triumph of high achievement, and who, at the worst, if he fails, at least he fails while daring greatly.[11]

Michelangelo's *David*

Years ago I went to a London exhibition that featured works by Michelangelo. Previously, I'd seen Michelangelo's famous marble statue *David* when I'd spent time in Florence, Italy, the statue's home. Standing in front of the marble figure, I found its beauty overwhelming and Michelangelo's genius palpable. The exhibit in London was very different from the one in Florence, and rather than displaying the artist's best-known work, it featured the drafts that *led* to his best-known work: the sketches that led to *David*.

The memory of one particular set of drawings of *David*'s arm has stayed with me. There were a few dozen drawings of the arm, one after another. The first drawing looked perfect to me. I wished I could do that. But clearly, Michelangelo wasn't satisfied with his first rendering, nor his tenth. He didn't feel that it was ready, yet. And given that he didn't have the benefit of computer technology to speed things up, he had to sketch the arm again and again until he was satisfied. It took Michelangelo dozens of attempts to produce the sketch that became the basis for *David*'s arm.

The Fear of Making a Mistake

How many of us consider ourselves to be perfectionists? Perfectionists are hypercritical of themselves, disparaging of mistakes, and terrified of failure. Nobody loves to err or fall down, but there is a difference between disliking failure and intensely fearing it. When we dislike failure, we are compelled to take precautions and work harder. Intense fear, on the other hand, is paralyzing and stops us from trying. The price that we pay for this paralysis is extremely high. When we put ourselves on the line and try, we risk failure; when we refrain from trying, we guarantee failure. Moreover, the failure that comes from trying is potentially a stepping-stone, an opportunity for learning and growing. In contrast, the failure that comes from not trying is a stumbling block, narrowing our opportunities for further progress.

In job interviews, people are often asked, "So, tell me about your greatest weakness," and they say, "Oh, my weakness is I'm a perfectionist." We're coached to give this answer in order to signal "I'm very responsible and reliable. You can trust me to do the job well." We think of these qualities as hidden strengths. But perfectionism comes with a dark side—the intense fear of failure that permeates every part of our life. This is what we need to overcome.

Perfectionism hurts us in many areas of our lives. For me, the biggest price I paid was in the context of my relationships. Because a perfectionist doesn't like to be wrong, I would often be defensive whenever my partner or a friend pointed to anything I perceived as a personal shortcoming. In arguments, I would automatically think (and sometimes say): *I am not wrong! You are!* Over the years, as I've learned to be more compassionate and more accepting of flaws and failures—seeing myself as a human being—I've become more open with others.

The way through is to be more forgiving of your imperfections. Self-compassion is just as important as compassion toward others.[12] When you're more forgiving, you are more open to learning from your mistakes and can make better decisions going forward. Even though failure hurts, and even though deviating from the straight and narrow may be challenging, it's an essential part of the process. You will find more success and happiness when you embrace failure rather than judge imperfection, forgive mistakes rather than chastise flaws.

The Growth Mindset

Another way to combat the fear of making mistakes is to develop a growth mindset.[13] The growth mindset is the belief that we are capable of change. Whether with regard to our mental skill, our ability to draw, to shoot a basket, to run a business, or to be in a relationship, it's the belief that our abilities are malleable and that we *can* improve. The opposite, the fixed mindset, is the belief that we're either born with an ability or not. We're either smart or we're not. We're either talented or ungifted. Our relationship is either absolutely great or damaged beyond repair. A fixed mindset doesn't allow for evolution.

How can you become more growth oriented? One way is to value process over outcome, effort over result. If you focus on effort and celebrate the process—including failures along the way—you're much more likely to create a growth mindset than if your primary focus is some end result. We can see this growth versus fixed mindset emerge from a very young age. To encourage a growth mindset in kids, shift what you praise. Don't emphasize the brilliance of the result or the achievement of the outcome. Instead focus on the effort. I have three kids, and with the three of them, I underplay outcomes. When they bring home a good grade, rather than saying, "I'm so glad you got an A" or, "You're so smart!" I say, "I'm really glad that you understand the material now. You invested the time and you learned." When they bring home a poor grade, rather than focusing on the result, I focus on what they learned and how they can learn further. I put the emphasis on the hard work, and on the process.

The most important thing as a parent is to lead by example. Share your failures with your children and tell them how you learned from those failures. There's a wonderful video of orchestra conductor Benjamin Zander of the Boston Philharmonic Youth Orchestra, where he teaches a teenager how to play the cello. Zander has a rule that every time his students make a mistake, he says, "How fascinating," celebrating the mistake, because each mistake is an opportunity for learning.

Psychological Safety

How can we help our loved ones, our colleagues, or others to learn, grow, and become antifragile? Research by Amy Edmondson from Harvard Business School has introduced the idea of psychological safety.[14] That is, having the sense of security that it's OK to fail within an organization or a group. For instance, if I'm a member of a team and I feel like it's acceptable for me to make mistakes, to admit I don't know something, and to be allowed to fail without the threat of being excluded, then there is psychological safety. Most organizations don't provide psychological safety or enough opportunity for failure. However, the ones that do have the happiest—and most effective—employees.

Google is one of the most sought-after employers in the world today, so people who work there are generally top performers. And yet, within Google there are teams that are highly productive and innovative, and teams that are less so. Recently, Google conducted research—and Google knows how to collect data—to identify what distinguishes the best from the rest.[15] They found that the top teams enjoyed high levels of psychological safety. Those teams felt that they had permission to fail, and hence, the latitude to experiment and innovate.

Does this mean that failure is always an option? That you as a manager or as a parent should give a blank check for failure? No. First, boundaries are critical when failure would be dangerous. It's why we direct children not to do certain things when it comes to an electrical outlet, for example, rather than encourage them to experiment with it and learn through trial and error. And second, failure is only useful when we are open to learn from the experience.

Let me share with you a brief story about James Burke, the legendary former CEO of Johnson & Johnson.[16] Early in his career, in the 1950s, Burke was a young and up-and-coming manager. He had just launched a new line of products for children, which turned out to be a "resounding failure." The company lost a lot of money. In the wake of this implosion, he was invited in to see the CEO, General Robert Wood Johnson II himself. Walking into his boss's office, Burke was certain that he was about to be fired. Instead, Johnson got up, extended his hand, and congratulated him. Burke was floored; he didn't know what was going on. General Johnson then went on to explain to Burke that it is only through experimenting and making mistakes that you learn how to do business. It's perfectly fine to make mistakes, as long as you reflect on them and apply what you learned.

James Burke not only didn't get fired, he went on to become an incredibly successful CEO at Johnson & Johnson, revered for seeing the company through its most difficult times and on to incredible growth during his tenure. Burke's journey demonstrates the importance of psychological safety—how room for error can become the space to develop antifragility and unleash our potential for growth.

Just as studying happiness is not about reaching a final destination but a process of becoming happier, intellectual wellbeing is not about determining final answers—its true value is in the process of exploring, discovering, and learning. And it is often a question that launches us on a quest.

The brilliant German poet Rainer Maria Rilke admonished himself and his readers to focus on the question rather than the answer, on the process rather than the outcome. In his book *Letters to a Young Poet*, Rilke wrote: "Be patient toward all that is unsolved in your heart and try to love the questions themselves . . . Live the questions now. Perhaps you will then gradually, without noticing it, live along some distant day into the answer."[17]

So that's what I urge you to do: Be patient with uncertainty. Ask your questions, and tap into your innate curiosity. Engage deeply with rich texts; choose one or two great books and indulge in them. Read and reread them, fulfilling your potential for deep learning, and through that, for success and happiness in other domains. Let go of perfection and allow yourself to fall down, and get up again.

Learn to fail or fail to learn. There is no other way.

THE SPIRE CHECK-IN

Intellectual Wellbeing

Go through the three steps of the SPIRE Check-In–ascribe, describe, and prescribe–focusing on intellectual wellbeing. Begin by reflecting on the following questions:

Are you learning new things?

Do you ask enough questions?

Do you engage in deep learning?

Are you failing enough?

Based on your reflections, determine the degree to which you experience intellectual wellbeing and then *ascribe* a score from 1 to 10, with 1 being very little or very infrequently, and 10 being very much or very often. After ascribing a score, in writing *describe* why you gave yourself that score. Then, *prescribe* a way to increase your score by just one point at first. For example, make a point of asking yourself and others more questions, pick up a book you value and reread it slowly, make a point of failing a little more (and when you do, celebrate it and yourself). Keep checking in with yourself once a week.

Chapter 4

—

Relational Wellbeing

Friendship doubles joy and cuts grief in half.
—Francis Bacon

What is the best predictor of happiness? This simple question looms large over data that has been collected for almost a century. Beginning in the late 1930s, researchers at Harvard embarked on a major long-term study, one that still continues today.[1] For generations, they followed two groups: a large cohort of students and members from the adjoining city. The researchers studied the participants over the course of their lives, using questionnaires, interviews, physiological assessments, and environmental measures. After all these decades, having collected quite literally millions of data points, researchers examined the facts in search of the most important component of a happy life.

What did they find? You guessed it. It's not money or accolades, material success or prestige. According to the research, the number one predictor of happiness is relationships—specifically, having socially supportive, intimate relationships. It's what amplifies the good times and buoys us through difficult ones. The interesting thing about this finding is that it didn't really matter who the relationships were with; for some people it was their romantic partner or a best friend, for others it was their extended family or close connections at work. Healthy relationships weren't the only factor important for happiness, but they were the most significant one.

The researchers asked another question as part of this study: What is the best predictor of health? Naturally, our physical health depends on many factors, but which one of these factors matters most? You guessed it again: relationships. Close relationships are the number one predictor of health *and* happiness. It may seem obvious that they matter a great deal, and yet it's all too easy to take our relationships for granted, to not invest as much in them, or to let them become less of a priority over time. Although most of us routinely claim that family relationships or friendships are the most important thing in our lives, often that doesn't match up with how much effort we put into cultivating them.

We also see evidence for the impact of social relationships when we look at the big picture of happiness levels around the globe.[2] An increasing number of countries are beginning to consider gross national happiness (GNH) as a measure of national health just as gross national product (GNP) or gross domestic product (GDP) are traditional measures of economic health. The United States does not have the happiest people in the world, despite its being the wealthiest country in the world. Nor does China, Japan, Singapore, South Korea, Germany, or the UK have the happiest people, even though they are among the most materially prosperous. Which places have the happiest populations in the world? Countries like Colombia, Denmark, Norway, Costa Rica, Israel, and Australia consistently rank among the highest. So why these places—Israel or Colombia, for instance, with their fair share of challenges? One reason: relationships. In all these countries, there is a great emphasis on social connection and social support, such as strong family bonds or a sense of solidarity with community. For example, in Denmark, 93 percent of the Danes are active members of social clubs. They have a place where they consistently interact with friends, where they support others and are themselves supported. In Israel and Colombia, time with family is considered important, even sacred.

"No man is an island," wrote poet John Donne. Our need for companionship is as real as our need for water and food. I'm not saying that intimate relationships lead to utopia or that the best ones are perfect. They can also bring challenges, especially as more of us are spending more time at home during the pandemic. When we are under the same roof, cooped up with the same few people day after day, there's going to be some friction. In this chapter, we'll talk about the importance of these conflicts, and not only how we can overcome them, but also how we can grow stronger from them. We'll also look at maintaining friendships while apart—how can relationships thrive when social distancing is a reality and social isolation is becoming the norm? Even in times of disorder, I hope to give you a few simple strategies you can follow to improve any relationship, whether it's with your romantic partner, family member, colleague, or friend.

Deep Relationships

Deep, meaningful, and intimate relationships play a crucial role in our becoming antifragile—our ability to grow stronger from hardship. And yet, cultivating these relationships in a world of quarantine, lockdowns, and physical distancing is very challenging. When our concern is genuine connection, online interactions are a poor substitute for the real thing.

Even before the coronavirus crisis, we were spending far too much time on social media, and the price we paid was extremely high. New York University sociologist Eric Klinenberg pointed out that "The greater the proportion of online interaction [versus face-to-face interaction] the lonelier you are."[3] Loneliness, as you might expect, erodes health and happiness. Among other things, it is associated with depression, heart disease, and a weaker immune system. As appealing as online interactions are, we sometimes need to disconnect in order to connect. Like so many things, social media is best consumed in moderation. Spending twenty minutes on social media may be fun; spending three hours a day will make you more prone to loneliness. Try having screen-free times and technology-free zones in your home: no computers allowed in the living room where the family sits together, no phones at the dinner table, and so on.

Cutting down on technology is absolutely vital for the next generation. Jean Twenge, a professor at San Diego State University, conducted extensive research exploring teenagers' mental health levels.[4] What she found was frightening. Between 2012 and 2017, levels of loneliness went up by close to 30 percent among teenagers.

Depression went up by more than 30 percent. Suicide rates went up by over 30 percent. This is all in just five years, constituting massive and unprecedented change. The question is, why? Why have rates of depression, loneliness, and suicide gone up so significantly in such a short period of time? Twenge combed through the data and identified the culprit: the rise of the smartphone. Kids were looking at their devices rather than at the person sitting next to them, spending much more time online than with people they cared about in real life.

Because of research like Eric Klineberg's on adults and Jean Twenge's on teenagers, in the past whenever I was asked how to cultivate relational wellbeing, my answer was simple and definitive: Get off of social media and go out and meet people. But this was before COVID-19. Today, things are different, and many of us no longer have the luxury to choose between virtual and in-person relationships. We're locked down in our homes, trying our best to keep our distance, and subject to physical isolation. In this new world, we have to relinquish old distinctions that no longer serve us and come up with new ones that do. Instead of thinking virtual versus physical, we have to think superficial versus deep.

Deep relationships *are* possible, even in a virtual reality. Personally, I felt tremendous disappointment when classes at Columbia University, where I was teaching when the coronavirus hit, shifted to online. It had taken me more than a month—and a handful of two-hour sessions—to feel like my class on happiness studies took the magical shift that I so crave when teaching, from superficial academic discussions to deep psychological conversations. When we went online, I feared this magic would be lost. And initially it was. To my surprise, however, within a couple of sessions the screen ceased to be a barrier to intimacy. The first steps in this new virtual territory were precarious, but as soon as one student and then another took the plunge and shared what was on their minds and hearts, others provided support and then themselves followed into the deep. Together we discovered that intimacy and depth are possible online.

In a world that has lost much of its old structures—where boundaries between work and home, in space and in time, are crumbling—we need to establish some new structures. And perhaps the most important structure in this new normal is regularly setting aside the time for deep, meaningful, heartfelt conversations. Ideally, these connections would be in-person—being together in the same home, or the same restaurant—hanging out and spending quality time with people we care about and who care about us. When that's not possible, we can use technology to make up for it and cultivate meaningful relationships no matter where we are. Just as deep learning is essential for intellectual wellbeing, deep conversations are necessary for relational wellbeing. Whether you go on a Zoom date with a friend or just hear each other's voices on the phone, take the time to authentically connect—to open up and share, to listen and support.

Cultivating Empathy

It's not just our mental health that has been radically affected since the onset of social media, but also our empathy. Social psychologist Sara Konrath compared levels of empathy across generations and found that among twenty-year-olds today levels are 40 percent lower than those of twenty-year-olds from twenty years ago.[5] Similarly, a study in the UK found that antisocial behavior doubled among high school students over the last twenty years. In other words, compassion has gone down significantly. And with that, bullying behavior has been on the rise.

Empathy—being able to understand and identify with what others are feeling—is the moral sentiment. Empathy is what ties us together, and when our ability to empathize decreases, it spells trouble for us as a society.[6] Why have levels of empathy gone down? One of the main reasons is because people are less often authentically and deeply interacting with one another.

Given the declining levels of empathy, calls abound for empathy education classes in schools, and while that would be a step in the right direction, alone it isn't enough. Let's say I want to learn to speak Vietnamese, so I enroll in classes. While my Vietnamese will certainly improve, it will improve much more if I go to Vietnam and immerse myself in the culture that speaks the language. The same is true for the language of empathy. We can learn about the importance of putting ourselves in other people's shoes by reading or taking a class. I might read *The Theory of Moral Sentiments* by Adam Smith or take a class on Ubuntu as an ethical construct. But the more effective method is to immerse myself in the place where empathy is "spoken." That is, to go wherever I can interact face-to-face with other people. Only through direct interactions can we sense what someone else might be experiencing and feeling. That's when we can laugh with someone; that's when we can cry together. That's when we might do something wrong and hurt someone and be affected by their reaction. And that's how empathy develops. Ideally, these interactions occur when children play side by side, or when we sit together in school or at work, unmediated by a screen. But if we have no other choice, then we have to—and can—do it virtually.

One silver lining of being stuck at home is that it has taught me to appreciate my relationships with family and friends and to value our time in one another's presence. I suspect the same is true for many of us. Hopefully this appreciation will translate into more time spent in intimate gatherings when these are possible again. It is when we interact closely with other people, whether with our loved ones or with strangers we've just met, that we develop more empathy, kindness, and compassion, as well as enjoy higher levels of physical and mental wellbeing. We become more ethical and more generous, healthier and happier.

The Power of Giving

In a time when we're more isolated than ever, how else can we meaningfully strengthen our relationships? No matter what your situation, one of the best ways to become more empathetic and alleviate feelings of loneliness is through giving.

In a joint study between the University of British Columbia and Harvard Business School, researchers demonstrated the power of giving.[7] For the first part of the study, the researchers brought in a group of people and measured their levels of happiness. Then they gave them each a nice sum of money and told them to spend it on themselves. So the subjects went on a shopping spree. The researchers measured their levels of happiness again. What do you think they found?

As a result of going shopping, the subjects' happiness levels went up significantly. The study continued and they brought the participants back to the lab one day later. Once again, they measured their levels of happiness. What do you think they found now? After twenty-four hours, happiness levels went right back down to where they were before. In other words, subjects experienced a high as a result of shopping, and then very quickly reverted to their previous state. So is the conclusion from this research that we need to go shopping every day? Not exactly.

In the second part of the study, the researchers brought in a different group of people, randomly selected, and measured their levels of happiness. They gave them the same amount of money and told them to go out and spend it. Only this time, the participants had to spend it on someone else. The participants came back to the lab afterward and again had their happiness assessed. Their levels of happiness went up by as much as the initial subjects' had. The next day, researchers measured their levels of happiness again, and what did they find? Although happiness levels did go down a little bit, they were still significantly higher than they were at base level. As it turns out, the act of giving continued to have a beneficial impact a week after the event.

When we give to others, we're also giving to ourselves. There's a great deal of research showing that giving is one of the best ways to not only increase happiness, but also to increase self-confidence. Giving can take us from helplessness to helpfulness, and consequently from hopelessness to hopefulness. The difference between sadness and depression is that depression is sadness without hope. Giving introduces hope. And as you become more hopeful, you become more capable, happier, and ultimately more successful.

English is my second language; my mother tongue is Hebrew. My favorite word in Hebrew is the word for give, *natan* (נ ת ן). Looking at the word, whether in Hebrew or Roman letters, do you notice something unusual about it? It's a palindrome. It is symmetrical, reading the same from right to left and left to right. That's no coincidence. There's a lot of wisdom in many of the ancient languages, and in the case of *natan*, research clearly demonstrates that when we give, we receive, often with interest. One of the best ways to cultivate strong, intimate relationships is to enter those relationships with the mindset and heartset of a giver.

What can we give? Anything. At merely thirteen years old, Anne Frank wrote in her diary "You can always, always give something, even if it is only kindness." We give when we do a chore for our partner unprompted, or surprise a friend. Actively listening to our children is a form of giving, as is sharing information with a colleague. As we'll see in Chapter 5, one of the most powerful happiness interventions is writing a gratitude letter. When you write a gratitude letter to another person—appreciating that person—you're giving. You're being kind. You're being generous. And when we give, we don't just increase other people's levels of happiness, we increase our own.

"Count That Day Lost"

Nineteenth-century author Mary Ann Evans, whose pen name was George Eliot, has written many wonderful books—perhaps best known is *Middlemarch*—including some beautiful poetry. This is one of her poems, "Count That Day Lost," about the importance of giving.

If you sit down at set of sun

And count the acts that you have done

And, counting, find

One self-denying deed, one word

That eased the heart of him who heard,

One glance most kind

That fell like sunshine where it went—

Then you may count that day well spent.

But if, through all the livelong day

You've cheered no heart, by yea or nay—

If, through it all

You've nothing done that you can trace

That brought the sunshine to one face—

No act most small

That helped some soul and nothing cost—

Then count that day as worse than lost.

According to Evans, a day when we bring sunshine to another, where we bring kindness, generosity, and love, that's a "day well spent." Whereas if we go through the day without having a positive impact on people's lives, then that day is "worse than lost." Now imagine if giving were the currency by which we measured our lives. If we evaluated how we are doing in terms of how generous and kind we are, by how much we spread joy, this world would be a much better place. Not just for those who benefit from our good deeds, but also for ourselves.

Give to Yourself, Too

Should we give, give, and give relentlessly? If you're the type of person who rushes to take care of everyone in your orbit, and meanwhile, you're low on fuel and on the verge of flaming out, know that it is possible to give too much of yourself. Psychologist Adam Grant, a professor at the University of Pennsylvania, led research into people's different approaches in the workplace. Along with his colleagues, Grant identified three general groups: the givers, the takers, and the matchers.[8] As their name suggests, the givers are those who give of their time, energy, and expertise freely. They are the nice employees, the helpful workers. Then there are the takers. What the givers give, the takers are eager to take—it's mostly all about them. They ask for favors and are reluctant to offer others the same. And then there are the matchers. Matchers have a quid pro quo philosophy—they give to others precisely as much as they think they received—and don't like seeing someone get more then they "deserve."

From a management perspective, you want to have givers in your organization. You want people who are generous, who teach, who help others, who are there for the team and who care about the organization. However, while the company may benefit from employees who are givers, what does it mean for the individuals themselves? Is it better to be a giver, a taker, or a matcher if you're concerned with long-term success? Does giving actually make you more successful? Does matching, because it's the most fair? Or is taking the way to go if you're all about success?

These are the questions that Grant and his fellow researchers addressed. They were able to group the organizations' employees by three levels of performance—top, middle, and bottom. Who tended to be the top performers? As it turns out, the most successful individuals in the organization were likely to be givers. They were disproportionately more successful. Who was in the middle? The takers and the matchers. So . . . who was left? Who did they find at the bottom? Givers! The surprising finding was that givers were more likely than takers or matchers to be among the best as well as the worst performers.

How can you distinguish the givers at the top from the givers at the bottom? The difference between them is that the top-performing givers also *give to themselves*. The givers in the lowest performing group, meanwhile, tend to forget about themselves—they give to the point of exhaustion, without attending to their own needs. And what they need in order to continue thriving is to think about helping themselves, too. This finding calls to mind the safety language that we often hear on airplane flights: Put on your oxygen mask first before assisting others.

The Dalai Lama spoke about this very idea: "Caring for others based only on your sacrifice doesn't last. Caring must also feed you."[9] This isn't a trivial idea for most Western people. Daniel Goleman, in his book *Destructive Emotions*, talks about the Dalai Lama's utter surprise at the fact that many people in the West have low self-esteem. How could people not like themselves? One of the reasons this is different in Tibet, the Dalai Lama suggested, is because of Tibetans' understanding of compassion. Words create worlds; the way we interpret particular concepts, which is often a product of our culture and environment, is important and often explains deeply rooted and subconscious psychological tendencies.

What is it that's so special about compassion? If I asked people in the West to define compassion, most would likely say that it means feeling sympathy for, and caring for, other people. The Dalai Lama says that in Tibetan, the word for compassion is *tsewa*, which means *compassion for self and compassion for others*.[10] Notably, it is the self first, and by extension others. Think about a series of concentric circles, in which you're at the center. You start with compassion for yourself, extend it to the people close to you, and then to others, and then to the whole world—but it begins with the self. We are all connected in this circle of life, in a web of compassion. In Eastern philosophical traditions (in contrast to Western traditions) there isn't a perceived split between one's self and others.

In Western philosophical traditions, a related split exists between selfish and selfless. Synonyms for the word *selfish* include *mean, ungenerous, narcissistic, greedy.* On the flip side, similar terms to *selfless* include *noble, generous, loving,* and *charitable.* From the time we learn language at a very young age, we're taught that thinking about the self (which includes being compassionate toward the self) is not moral. But that's not quite right—why is *my* self less worthy than *other* selves? —nor is it sustainable: Those who don't take care of their own needs will ultimately be left with nothing to give to themselves or to others. Instead of seeing giving to others as selfless and giving to oneself as selfish, we can think about healthy giving as *selful. Selfulness* is about taking care of others and of oneself.

What could selfulness look like? If a colleague were to ask me for help with their project, I could simply say, "I'd be happy to help you, but I need to finish this assignment first." At home, I can say, "Kids, I'll be with you after this workout is done," or, "Sweetheart, I will be with you tomorrow, but right now I just need some me time." And that's OK! Taking care of yourself doesn't make you a bad person. On the contrary, in the long haul, we're most likely to help and contribute, to be kind and generous toward others, when we also pay attention to our own needs. In the words of Hillel, one of the great Jewish sages who lived more than two thousand years ago, "If I'm not for myself, who will be for me? But if I'm only for myself, who am I? And if not now, then when?" Our world needs selful people, now more than ever.

Building Children's Resilience

During times of general upheaval, parents feel as though it is their duty to provide their children with a perfect role model, one that will consistently function as a stable pillar of support to lean on. *This is no time for weakness*, they think; *I have to be strong for my kid*. What do we do, though, when we're going through a crisis and are feeling weak, anxious, frustrated, sad, or angry? How do we manage our emotions in front of our kids when we know that our distress will further add to theirs?

We first need to keep in mind that it's fine for children to see us struggling, even if that adds to their struggles. Our impulse as parents is to protect them, to hide rather than reveal our emotional turmoil. But witnessing parents experience sadness or anxiety or anger—in moderation—is necessary for kids' healthy development. More generally, as parents we should accept that being a perfect role model for our children is not only impossible, it is also undesirable.

Nearly seventy years ago, Donald Winnicott, a British child psychologist, introduced one of the most important concepts regarding parenting: "the good enough mother."[11] What does it mean? Winnicott recognized that many parents want to be the perfect caregivers who are always attentive. When the child cries, the parent immediately provides comfort; when the child encounters challenges, the parent is right there to help. Winnicott pointed out that this is not what children need. What children need are *good enough parents*. If parents are not one hundred percent attentive to their children, whether it's because they are busy, upset, or working and need some time alone, that's not a bad thing. Through this lack of attention, children learn self-regulation; in contrast, when parents are always available, children don't learn to deal with difficulties on their own. Our ultimate goal as parents is to raise independent children. After all, parents cannot always be by their children's side throughout their life. Children must be given opportunities to cope from the time they are born. The good enough parent is then much closer to what a child needs than is a so-called perfect parent.

Being "good enough" also means it's perfectly fine if your children occasionally see you when you're upset. You may even talk to them about it; you can hold them so that they feel secure, and say "I'm upset right now" or "I'm just drained." You can be loving and caring while conveying to them that everything is not OK. In fact, it can be liberating for kids to hear it from you, because they feel that way sometimes as well. By giving yourself permission to be human, it gives them that permission, too.

Even if they do see you fly off the handle, it's not the end of the world. They also see you afterward when you recover, which is reassuring. You can apologize to them if you've said something in your emotional state that you shouldn't have, or that you regret. Kids don't need perfect role models; they need good enough human beings. One of the beautiful elements of parenting is that you are not just teaching other people, you're also growing yourself. A parent who is learning is the best role model that a child can have.

Many parents, understandably, have worried about the effects of the pandemic on their kids. One of the biggest challenges that we're facing as parents—and when I say *we*, I mean many people in wealthier, developed countries, and not everyone out there by any stretch—is that we've been making the lives of our children too easy, out of a sense of wanting to protect them, and also because we can. It's natural that we want to give our children the best. But research by Suniya Luther at Columbia University shows that many children from well-to-do families are suffering from psychological distress, such as anxiety, depression, or substance abuse, because of this trap of luxury.[12] Life is about learning how to deal with things not going according to plan. Being confronted with obstacles, though inconvenient or painful in the short term, can be beneficial.

Let me share with you an experience I had that brought this idea to the fore in my life. When David, my eldest son, was three years old, his favorite toy was a tiny Superman doll. He would play with it throughout the day and put it next to him on his pillow before he went to sleep. One day my wife and I picked up David from daycare and went home—we lived on the tenth floor of an apartment building. We went into the elevator; my wife and I were talking to each other, while David was talking to little Superman. The doors opened at our floor, and as we stepped out of the elevator, David accidentally dropped Superman. This Superman did not fly. This Superman fell right into the narrow gap between the doors, all the way down the elevator shaft. Gone. Not even Mom or Dad could get him back.

David began to bawl. As we hugged David to reassure him, I was about to open my mouth, but as is very often the case, my wife knew what I was about to say before I said it, and she stopped me. I was about to say, "David, don't worry. We'll get you another Superman doll. We can get you a hundred Superman dolls." As we went inside, David ran to his room and continued to cry. I said to my wife, "Why did you stop me? Listen to our son crying!" And she said to me: "Tal, do not deprive David of the opportunity to learn to deal with hardship."

Do not deprive David of the opportunity to learn to deal with hardship—it's one of the most important parenting lessons that I've ever learned. She was absolutely right: this is how children (and adults) learn resilience, resourcefulness, and creativity. This is how children learn flexibility, or, more accurately, fluidity. The *Tao Te Ching* talks about the ideal for humans as being like water for many reasons, and one of them is because water flows. "What is soft is strong," wrote Lao Tzu.

If we put our exercise equipment on the easiest setting, with little or no resistance, it makes for a cushy workout, but we won't get any stronger. There will be no antifragility. On the other end of the spectrum, if we struggle too much, we can get hurt and injured. But if we're allowed to struggle sometimes, in moderation with recovery, we are able to grow. It's the same in life, and as parents, many of us swoop in to rescue our children too quickly. Maria Montessori, one of the greatest educators in history, emphasized in her teaching that we must not do for a child what the child can do for himself or herself.[13] That doesn't mean not doing anything for young children, of course; when they can't handle something on their own, parents should be there for them. However, as much as possible, we should minimize the help we offer and instead allow them to help themselves.

Speaking to his graduating students at Harvard Business School, professor Clayton Christensen shared this parting message: "The challenges your children will face serve an important purpose. They help them hone and develop capabilities they need to succeed throughout their lives. Coping with a difficult teacher, failing at a sport, learning to navigate the complex social structure of cliques in school—all those things become courses in the school of experience."[14] Now, we can add to the list coping with remote schooling, social distancing, and canceled activities that they'd been looking forward to. Children learn from challenges, and gaining experience in overcoming difficulties early on makes it easier for them to handle problems and become role models for others when they grow up.

Love and Conflict

Conflicts are inevitable in any committed relationship, and during stressful periods they are more frequent than in normal times. It's not easy to be with the same person in a small apartment or the same few people at home for long periods. At the same time, with this challenge also comes a real opportunity. Conflict, it turns out, is important—even necessary—for love to grow.

Back in 1841, Ralph Waldo Emerson published an essay on friendship. In a friend, we should not be looking for "a mush of concession," he wrote—in other words, a person who will agree with everything that we say. Rather, "Let him be to thee forever a sort of beautiful enemy, untamable, devoutly revered, and not a trivial convenience to be soon outgrown and cast aside."[15] I love that phrase, *beautiful enemy*. A beautiful enemy is someone who challenges you, who pushes you, who helps you in your "apprenticeship to the truth," in the words of Emerson. When you're with a beautiful enemy, things are sometimes difficult, though the potential for growth is ever present. Instead of "trivial convenience," you experience meaningful inconvenience; rather than ease that numbs, you experience conflict that nurtures.

We find this idea of a beautiful enemy early on in the first book of the Bible. In Genesis, God says, "It is not good that the man should be alone. I will make a helpmeet for him." *Help meet* is a direct translation from the Hebrew words *ezer k'enegdo*, which literally means "help as opposition." In the English version, *meet* refers to competition, as in an athletic meet. In other words, helpmeet is a partner who challenges you to grow. Learning to see our partner as a beautiful enemy, as a helpmeet, can help us reframe conflicts within our relationships: Rather than seeing discord as a dangerous, dark spot that is to be averted at all cost, we can see it as a valuable opportunity for personal and interpersonal growth.

Dr. David Schnarch, author of *Passionate Marriage*—a book that has radically changed my life—highlights the significant role conflicts play in the evolution of every successful relationship. Schnarch suggests that within every relationship, no matter how amazing it is, couples will invariably reach a gridlock. A gridlock is an extreme conflict. It's not one of those everyday arguments where we fight, make up, make love, and then everything is great again. A gridlock is a fundamental disagreement over one of our core values, which we've just discovered is in opposition to an equally deep-seated belief within our partner. Couples are generally exempt from a gridlock during the honeymoon phase of their relationship, but within three years or so, it invariably strikes and usually revolves around one of the following four topics:

1. **Children.** What approach to discipline should we take? Should we be lenient or should we be more forceful? What limits are we setting? What education should our kids receive? What role should religion play in their upbringing?

2. **Money.** What should we spend money on? Should we make this major purchase at this point? Does one partner feel the other is buying too many things, or not contributing enough? Can we afford this? Are we saving enough?

3. **Sex.** How often are we having sex? Does one partner think it's too much or not enough? What kind of sex? Is the sex we're having too kinky or too vanilla? Should we open our relationship or remain exclusive, try polyamory or stick with monogamy?

4. **Extended family.** Should we invite our in-laws over once a week? Should we never invite them? How much should we involve the rest of the family in our decision making? How often should we attend family reunions? Weekly? Never?

When we reach a gridlock, one of three things can happen. The first common outcome is a breakup, separation, or divorce. Between 40 and 50 percent of marriages end in divorce. *I thought we were perfect for each other, but if we can disagree on something so important to me, evidently we're not.* This is why divorce levels commonly spike four to seven years into marriage; couples encounter their first gridlock and consequently think their differences are irreconcilable.

The second thing you can do after a gridlock is stay together, but not really be together. Meaning, you stay together for any number of external reasons—out of habit, or because of religion, or for the kids, or for financial reasons. But emotionally, you've parted ways.

Option number three is to grow together as a result of the gridlock. You argue, you disagree, you clash. And then after a while—and it could be after a week, a month, or six months—both of you emerge better off individually and as a couple. How do you get to option three, the antifragile option, and go through the gridlock successfully? First of all, you struggle. Second, as you struggle, you hold on to yourself rather than conform, respectfully express your needs and wants rather than dismiss them. Third, as you're holding on to yourself, you hold on to the relationship by staying put and through it all seeking to understand your partner's needs and wants. The key is not to make each other feel good—to validate and seek validation—but instead "to know and to be known." It is by getting to know each other better—weaknesses and strengths, fears and fantasies—that intimacy is forged. And with intimacy comes love, passion, and compassion.

Genuinely striving to know and to be known means taking a risk. Let's say you've had an issue with your in-laws and, while you really don't want to talk about it with your partner because of how much he cares about his parents, it's hurting you. Eventually, you bring it up with as much empathy as you can. While it may lead to a painful conflict, the alternative is guaranteed unhappiness. In the early stages of a relationship, you can avoid talking about uncomfortable topics; you're sustained by the excitement of novelty. But after a while, that's just not enough, and sweeping things under the rug doesn't solve anything. On the contrary, as the issue festers, you eventually fall apart, and the relationship disintegrates.

Not every gridlock can be resolved and lead to a deeper relationship. Some couples are too far apart on certain issues and just not meant to be together—and that's fine. However, in most cases, gridlocks present important opportunities for learning, for us to become better individuals, and for our relationship to grow. When we communicate openly, with the real intention of making our relationship work, we usually find a solution and overcome the gridlock—whether it's through one partner convincing the other, reaching a compromise, or becoming creative and finding a win for both partners.

Experiencing conflicts, whether minor disagreements or full-on gridlocks, helps build your relationship's immune system, whereas in a sterile environment where conflicts are avoided, you don't develop critical antibodies. So if you want your relationship to survive, let alone thrive, you don't really have a choice—you have to work through challenges. Make it a point to open up to your partner, to address issues that are important to you, because when you do, ultimately you benefit, your partner benefits, as does your relationship.

Understanding David Schnarch's idea that disagreement does not equal incompatibility transformed my own relationship. It happened when my wife and I had been together for a decade. I thought we were meant for each other, until we reached a gridlock, and then I was suddenly overcome with fear and anxiety. *What's happening? I was certain that she is the love of my life, yet we disagree so strongly about something that is so important to both of us. Is this the beginning of the end?* Then I read *Passionate Marriage* and I realized, no. There's nothing wrong with our relationship; there's everything right with it. It's simply going through a natural evolution. As Schnarch writes, "Marriage operates at much greater intensity and pressure than we expect—so great, in fact, couples mistakenly assume it's time for divorce when it's really time to get to work." We put in the work and were able to grow through that gridlock and a few others that came after. Gridlocks are scary because they leave us open, prone, vulnerable. However, once you've gone through a major conflict, later ones are easier (albeit not easy), because there is less fear associated with it; you already know that you can survive it. You have hope.

There is no guaranteed path through any conflict, but if you create the conditions for openness and authenticity, resolution is more likely to happen. Here are some additional strategies to keep in mind as you enter conflict, regardless of its magnitude.

Reflect. It helps to just take a step back from the relationship to reflect—whether it's to consult with someone or to write about it in your journal. Remember, the givers at the top also give to themselves. One way to do that is to say, "I need time by myself to regroup, think, figure things out."

Listen and empathize. Put aside your own arguments and preconceptions for a few minutes or hours, and really hear and be open to what your partner is saying. Resist the urge to distract yourself from the conversation or interrupt with your side of the story, and don't dismiss their concerns as unimportant. A recent study published in the *Journal of Family Psychology* showed that "attentive listening while the other partner expressed stress was linked with better dyadic coping behaviors and higher relationship satisfaction."[16] Genuinely listening and making an effort to understand your partner's viewpoint is a sign of empathy (an effect) and a further reinforcer of empathy (a cause).

Find ways to get to yes. University of Washington psychologist John Gottman, one of the world's leading researchers on relationships, interviewed hundreds of couples and analyzed their conversations. The data clearly shows that respectful, positive conversations are at the core of marital success: "It sounds simple, but in fact you could capture all of my research findings with the metaphor of a saltshaker. Instead of filling it with salt, fill it with all the ways you can say yes, and that's what a good relationship is. 'Yes,' you say, 'that is a good idea.' 'Yes, that's a great point, I never thought of that.' . . . In a partnership that's troubled, the saltshaker is filled with all the ways you can say no." Gottman further demonstrates that the best relationships enjoy a 5:1 positivity ratio, meaning that for every one disagreement or conflict, angry exchange, or disappointment, there are five positives—a compliment or a loving text message, perhaps; a smile, a hug, or a kiss; a romantic walk on the beach, lovemaking, or an intimate dinner. So while conflicts are inevitable— and, as we've seen, important—we need to complement those with a significantly higher number of positive experiences.

Be kind. Being kind is an important means of raising the positivity ratio. It sounds so simple to be kind, doesn't it? But how often do we find ourselves reaching for an insult, treating our partner with hostility? More than anything, a relationship thrives on basic courtesy and respect, and yet so many people take the liberty of being rude or hostile toward those who are closest to them. This is unfair to the partner and harmful to the relationship. What's something you can do to be kind to your partner even if you are in the midst of a disagreement? That one kind gesture is often enough to defuse tension so you can work toward a solution.

Take care of yourself. Exercise regularly, meditate, get a good night's sleep, take time to listen to music, indulge in reading—or do anything else that will replenish your resources and help you recover. You may be wondering *How are these choices related to relationships?* They are very deeply related in that they can be the catalyst for an upward spiral. Take exercise, for example: Exercising releases the feel-good chemicals in the brain. When I feel good about myself, I'm likely to be more patient with my partner and with my children. Similarly, when I meditate and give myself time for recovery, I become more open, more generous, and kinder to my loved ones, and hence my relationships are going to be better. I start with the self and expand outward.

David Schnarch describes emotionally committed relationships as "people growing machines." This applies to relationships between children and parents, as well as between partners. Growing, however, does not happen by default, and especially during stressful times we see many relationships and the individuals within those relationships wither. For our relationships to be antifragile and flourish no matter what, we need to allow space for conflict and positivity, knowing and being known, listening and expressing, giving to the other and giving to ourselves.

THE SPIRE CHECK-IN:

Relational Wellbeing

Go through the three steps of the SPIRE Check-In—ascribe, describe, and prescribe—focusing on relational wellbeing. Begin by reflecting on the following questions:

Do you spend quality time with your family and friends?

Are your relationships deep?

Do you take care of yourself?

Are you a giver?

Based on your reflections, determine the degree to which you experience relational wellbeing and then *ascribe* a score from 1 to 10, with 1 being very little or very infrequently, and 10 being very much or very often. After ascribing a score, in writing *describe* why you gave yourself that score. Then, *prescribe* a way to increase your score by just one point at first. Examples may include putting time aside to be with your loved ones, being a little kinder and giving a little more, refraining from helping when you don't have to, appreciating your beautiful enemies, and so on. Keep checking in with yourself once a week.

Chapter 5

—

Emotional Wellbeing

Your joy is your sorrow unmasked.
And the selfsame well from which your laughter
rises was oftentimes filled with your tears.
And how else can it be?
The deeper that sorrow carves into your being,
the more joy you can contain.

—Kahlil Gibran, *The Prophet*

Years ago when I was a graduate student, I had just started teaching my first class on positive psychology and had only eight students enrolled. Initially. Then two of them dropped out, which officially left me with . . . a broken ego. One day, I was having lunch in one of the undergraduate dorms when a student I knew, who was not in my class, came over. He said, "Tal, may I join you?" And I said, "Sure."

So he sat down and said, "I hear you're teaching a class on happiness," and I replied, "That's right, it's about positive psychology."

He quickly added, "You know, my roommate is taking your class, so you'd better watch out."

"Watch out? Why?" I asked.

"Because," he replied, "if I ever see you unhappy, I'm going to tell him."

I mentioned that conversation the following day in class when I addressed my students, all six of them: "You know, the last thing in the world that I want you to think is that I'm always happy, or that by the end of this year you will experience a constant high." The assumption behind this student's remark—that a happy life must be devoid of sadness or any other unpleasant emotion—is a common one. In fact, there are only two kinds of people who don't experience painful emotions such as sadness, anger, frustration, envy, or anxiety. The first kind are the psychopaths. Psychopaths do not experience the full range of human emotions; that's their limitation. The second group of people who do not experience painful emotions are dead.

So if you are experiencing painful emotions, it's a good sign. It means 1) you're not a psychopath and 2) you're alive.

Not long after that lunch with my student's roommate was when I first came up with the idea of the permission to be human. Since then, I've come to look at it as a fundamental pillar of a happier life. Permission to be human is about allowing yourself to feel any and all emotions, however painful they may be. Giving yourself this permission is to acknowledge, *I feel this right now, and that's fine* or as Demi Lovato put it: "It's OK not to be OK."

Giving yourself the permission to be human might be about letting yourself feel the fear of contracting the coronavirus. Or the anxiety that you've been laid off from your job. The worry that your kids are falling behind in school. The heartbreak of a loved one's diagnosis. The frustration of not being able to travel. The uncertainty of when the next wildfire or hurricane might strike your community. The sadness of having lost touch with a friend. The jealousy of how well your ex seems to be doing right now. The annoyance that, for the umpteenth time, no one seems to know how to load the dishwasher in your household except you. The anger that, whatever it is, *you didn't sign up for this.* Rather than hold back, it is better to accept the emotions and let them flow.

We do not generally treat all of our emotions equally; we welcome the joyful emotions but attempt to bar entry to those on the painful side of the spectrum. The very fact that painful emotions are commonly referred to as *negative* emotions points to the pervasive and harmful attitude toward them.

Part of the problem, especially in today's world where social media reigns supreme, is that we assume everyone else is having an amazing life all the time. We believe everyone is excelling and coping just fine, if not experiencing near-constant elation, while we're the only outliers who can't seem to keep it together. And we don't want to appear abnormal, so we hide our sadness, and we hide our anxiety and fear. *How are you doing? I'm good, you?* Our determination to don the mask of happiness is ultimately self-defeating—we're contributing to a great deception that leads to our great depression.

When my first child, David, was born, our pediatrician offered some valuable advice. Hours after the delivery the pediatrician walked into our hospital room to check on my wife and the baby. After making sure we were doing fine, he said to us, "Over the next few months you're going to experience a whole range of emotions, often to the extreme. You're going to feel joy and awe, frustration and anger, happiness and irritation. This is normal. We all go through it."

It was the best advice I received those first few months of being a parent. Why? Because after about a month cooped up with a newborn, I started to feel some envy toward David. For the first time since my wife and I had been together, here was someone who was getting more of her attention. No matter how exhausted and sleep-deprived and drained I was, no matter how much I need-ed her, his needs came first. Had the pediatrician not had that conversation with us, I would have thought to myself, *Wow, Tal, what a horrible dad you are. You're a bad person. Envious of your own son? That's disgusting.* But I heard the doctor's voice in the back of my mind, giving me the permission to be human, saying, *This is normal. We all go through it.* Because of his advice, I was able to allow that envy to flow through me, and it did. Five minutes later, the emotion had passed, and I was open to experience the love I felt and continue to feel toward my son.

Rejecting Emotions Makes Them Stronger

There is a paradox at play here: When we reject pain-ful emotions, they only intensify. We reject them again; they grow stronger and gnaw at us more deeply. Where-as when we accept and embrace painful emotions, they don't overstay their welcome. They visit and then leave just as they came.

Let's take grief, for example, arguably the strongest of painful emotions. Research suggests that people who go through grief fall roughly into two groups. One group comprises those who are considered to be tough. Following a loss, they decide, "I'm going to be strong. I'm going to get through this. I won't let this get to me." They put on a brave face, pick themselves up by their bootstraps, and go on. The other group, those who are considered softer and less tough, might say, "This is the worst thing that's ever happened to me, and I don't know how I'm going to get through it." They cry, they talk about it, and they experience their emotions. They break down.

When we look at the two groups from the outside, we might look at the first group and think, *Wow, they are holding up so well.* We might look the second group and think, *I'm worried and just hope that they will be OK and make it through.* But a year or more later, what the research suggests is that the second group is likely to be in a much better place than the first group. The second group gave themselves the permission to be human and allowed the natural process of grief to take its course.

Why does it work this way, whether for grief or anxiety or envy? Why do painful emotions subside when embraced, and intensify when rejected? Here's a little experiment. For the next ten seconds, do *not* think of a pink elephant. You know the one I'm talking about, Dumbo with the big ears? That pink elephant? Well, do not think of a pink elephant for two more seconds.

My strong hunch is that you thought of a pink elephant. Why? Because when a phrase is repeated over and over again, we think about it. And when we hear *do not think of it,* when we try to suppress the thought, it makes us more likely to continue to visualize it. That's part of our nature. This phenomenon, described by psychologist Daniel Wegner as part of his ironic process theory, applies to painful emotions as well.[1] When we attempt to reject painful emotions, they grow stronger and persist longer.

Our emotions are a phenomenon as natural as the law of gravity. Imagine you wake up every morning and say to yourself, *I've had it with the law of gravity. I refuse to accept gravity!* What will happen as a result? Well, first of all, you may fall down. And if you live in a tall building or enjoy hiking mountains, you may not survive for long. But, even if you did survive, you would lead a life of constant frustration. So, naturally, we don't reject the law of gravity. We accept it. We embrace it, we even play games with it. Imagine the javelin throw competition or the high jump event at the Olympics without gravity? Meaningless.

Yet we don't treat painful emotions in the same way. When we ignore the fact that emotions are as much a part of human nature as the law of gravity is part of physical nature, we pay a high price for that rejection.

When I started to teach, my biggest challenge was that I'm an introvert. I get very nervous in front of a large audience, real or virtual. In the beginning, when gearing up for a class I would say to myself, *Tal, don't be anxious! Don't be nervous!* What do you think happened? I would become even more nervous. Heart palpitations. Sweaty palms and forehead. Mind racing. More pink elephants flying around. Whereas when I started to give myself the permission to be human—when I accepted the anxiety, rather than tried to push it away—those nervous emotions eventually dissipated instead of escalating. Before a lecture I am still a little nervous, but instead of saying to myself, *Tal, don't be nervous*, I say to myself, *Wow, I'm so grateful that I'm not a psychopath and I'm alive*. The anxiety, more often than not, loses its hold on me and is replaced by excitement.

Viktor Frankl's theory of paradoxical intentions takes Wegner's ironic process theory a step further: Not only should we not interfere with the flow of painful emotions, we should encourage them. For example, if we don't want to feel nervous, we should tell ourselves, *Be more anxious. This is not enough nervous energy. Come on, more anxiety!* What's interesting is that by urging on the anxiety—which is really, again, about giving ourselves the permission to feel it—the anxiety is likely to weaken.

There's another paradox at work as well. It's not just that painful emotions intensify when we reject or avoid them—it's also that we fail to experience the full range of pleasurable emotions. All of our feelings, whether plea-surable or painful, flow through the same pipeline. If I reject the painful emotions, if I try to restrain and stop them, I'm also obstructing the free flow of pleasurable ones. As a result, I'm not allowing myself to experience my full range of emotions. If I block the envy, I'm also inadvertently blocking the love. If I restrict anxiety, I'm also restricting excitement. If I suppress sadness, I'm also impeding the free flow of joy. Painful and pleasurable emotions are two ends on one continuum; two sides of the same coin. In the words of Golda Meir, Israeli prime minister from 1969 to 1974, "Those who don't know how to weep with their whole heart don't know how to laugh, either."

We can think about suffering occurring on two levels. The first level is the natural and automatic experience of a painful emotion like anger, sadness, frustration, or anxiety, which we all feel from time to time. This can happen because of a myriad of events that trigger a painful emotional reaction, whether in anticipation of an upcoming presentation or a dangerous situation, as a result of loss of income or of a loved one, and so on. But there is a second level of suffering, which is inflicted when you fight that first level of suffering. When you say to yourself, *I shouldn't be angry!* or *I shouldn't be anxious!* or *I shouldn't envy!*, fighting the emotion only adds to the suffering. The *Tao Te Ching* says that if we are to live a fulfilling life we need to adhere to the way of nature, which is to flow with things rather than fight them.

Although the first level is an inevitable part of being human, when it comes to the second level of suffering, you have a choice. If you accept the emotion, then you exempt yourself from the denial that compounds the pain. By giving yourself the permission to be human, you fortify your ability to deal with hardship, you become more flexible in the face of painful emotions, and you open yourself up to more pleasurable emotions. You become more antifragile.

There are three specific ways of giving ourselves the permission to be human when facing painful emotions.

> **1. Cry.** Shed tears. Allow those floodgates to open. Simply close yourself up in your room and sob if that's what you feel like doing. Crying has been shown to be self-soothing; it releases feel-good chemicals like oxytocin and certain opioids that help in alleviating sadness and stress.[2]

2. Talk about painful emotions. Find yourself a Zoom buddy, or if you have someone living under the same roof as you to delve deep with, by all means. Express rather than suppress, share rather than try to hold it all in. Just talking about difficulties or challenges we're facing—whether with a trusted friend or with a therapist—helps us release tension and feel better.[3]

3. Write about the emotions. Take ten minutes or longer to journal about a difficult experience that you went through or are going through. Write about what you felt and what you are feeling, what you thought about then and what is going through your mind right now. You don't need to worry about grammar, sentence structure, or even whether or not you make sense. This is for your eyes only, so just write, free associate, whatever comes to mind and heart.

Psychologist James Pennebaker, a professor at the University of Texas, has demonstrated the profound impact of keeping a journal.[4] In Pennebaker's study, he had participants spend twenty minutes each day for four days writing about difficult experiences. Pennebaker measured many outcomes, including the subjects' anxiety levels. So what happened? Initially, when the participants were exposed to this journaling exercise, their anxiety levels increased. This was likely because they were bringing up events that took place in the past and that may have been parked somewhere in the subconscious. At first when Pennebaker saw these results, he was concerned that he was harming his subjects. But very quickly within the week, the participants' anxiety levels began to go down. Then they dropped to below the level where they started off. They sustained this drop even *a year later.* Those eighty minutes of intervention had a lasting positive impact on wellbeing.

I encourage you to take the time to keep a journal and write about your own difficult experiences. And if your journal gets repetitive? That's not a bad thing! Rest assured that even if you find yourself continually recording similar emotions, you are making progress. Think of it this way: How do you learn how to play the piano? How do you get better? Through practice, through repetition. You don't say to yourself, *OK, I'm going to sit down and try playing this difficult Rachmaninoff piece, but only once.* To fully understand the piece, to process it, you have to play it again and again. Similarly, sometimes you have to write about a difficult experience a number of times before you fully process it and understand what it is that you are going through.

In those confusing and chaotic weeks as we underwent lockdown in March 2020, isolating ourselves at home in response to the initial wave of coronavirus, I found a great deal of comfort in poetry. We introduced a few rituals in our household to get us through the difficult time; one was that every night we read a poem together. Early on we read "The Guest House" by Rumi, the thirteenth-century Sufi poet. In the poem, Rumi urges us to invite in any and all emotions and thoughts, just as we would welcome guests into our house, with an open heart and an open mind: "Be grateful for whatever comes."

Reading a poem can be a wonderfully comforting ritual, either together as a family or on your own. Poetry is an especially relevant medium for reflection during hard times because it presents things in unfiltered, deliberate language. It's about raw experiences, raw emotions.

In order to experience true happiness, we must first allow in unhappiness. The permission to be human is the foundation of building a happier life, no matter what.

Active Acceptance

Accepting your full range of human emotions is not an invitation to embrace resignation. That is, it's not about throwing up your hands and saying, "Well, I'm experiencing sadness and anger now, and that's all I can do. Sucks to be me." Rather, I encourage you to take the approach of *active acceptance*.

Active acceptance is about embracing the emotion and then choosing the most appropriate course of action. There is nothing wrong with experiencing painful emotions, just as there is nothing wrong with the law of gravity. Both are natural phenomena. The question is, what do we do about these natural phenomena? Do we resign ourselves to gravity and just fall down, or do we create ladders, bridges, airplanes? Do we succumb to a painful emotion, or do we choose an appropriate course of action?

Ultimately, action trumps emotion; what we do matters more than what we feel. Envying my child or my best friend, for example, doesn't make me a bad father or a bad friend. Envy may not be pleasant, but there is nothing immoral about feeling it; it simply is. However, if I were to act on that envy and hurt my son or hurt my friend, that is an entirely different story.

Part of the paradox that I introduced above—that painful emotions intensify when rejected—is that when we reject painful emotions they are more likely to control us, whereas when we accept our emotions we have more control over our subsequent actions. People who reject feeling fear are less likely to act courageously. People who reject the fact that they may feel anger toward others are ultimately more likely to blow up in fury. On the other hand, people who accept their fear are more likely to stand up and take bold action: Courage is not about *not* having fear, but about *having* fear and going ahead anyway. Those who accept their anger because they're human are more likely to act generously and benevolently toward other people.

Let's say you are feeling anxiety over the coronavirus or another health condition. If you simply think to yourself, *I shouldn't be anxious*, or *Don't worry*, well, you know what's going to happen. The worry and anxiety will rise, and could in time become an all-consuming panic. Whereas if you acknowledge, *I'm anxious and worried about this virus*, or simply, *I'm human*, and let yourself experience the emotion, then you can choose the most appropriate course of action.

You Are Not Your Emotion

Learning to observe painful emotions that we're experiencing is an important element of giving ourselves the permission to be human, and consequently, a key to emotional healing. Through observation, we learn to separate ourselves from whatever it is that we're feeling, and we shift from believing that *I am the emotion* to *I am having an emotion*. By looking at the emotion just as we would look at an object, we realize that just as we are not a flame or a breath or a stone, we are not an emotion.

This is no trivial matter or mere semantics. When talking about emotions, the fact that we merge who we are with what we feel—as in *I am sad* or *I am envious*—makes it more challenging to simply let go of the emotion. With a change in perspective—from *I am sad* to *I have sadness*, from *I am envious* to *I have envy*—it becomes much easier for us to break free of the emotion because we are not fused with it. We are not one with it, and therefore letting go of the emotion does not entail letting go of who we are.

As I discussed in the previous chapter on relationships, words create worlds: Our language impacts the way we think, feel, and act. It is important for us to change our language so that it becomes clear that *I am not my emotion* but rather that *I have an emotion*. After all, do I think to myself that *I am headache* when my head hurts? Just as *I have a headache*, I also have sadness or envy or any other emotion.

When observing an emotion that we're experiencing, what exactly do we focus on? An emotion is associated with thoughts (a cognitive component) and sensations (a physical component). Anxiety, for example, generates physical experiences, like a tight sensation in your throat, a knot in your belly, or tension in your shoulders or lower back. The sum total of the cognitive thoughts and the physical sensations is what we call the emotion.

In his coauthored book *The Mindful Way Through Depression*, Oxford University psychologist Mark Williams writes about observing the physical sensation associated with psychological dis-ease: "With the shift from trying to ignore or eliminate physical discomfort to paying attention with *friendly curiosity*, we can transform our experience."[5] Friendly curiosity is about not fighting or turning away from the sensation, but rather standing apart from it and observing it. It's looking at the physical manifestation of the emotion—the tight sensation in your throat or the knotted belly—as you would look at a work of art, or a dog playing, or a river flowing, and saying to yourself something like *Oh wow, look at that, how interesting!* This doesn't mean that the emotional experience is not painful, but only that you remain with the hurt and observe it with an open mind and heart. You then realize that you are the observer; the sensation is the observed. In other words, you are not the sensation—by observing it you distance and differentiate yourself from it.

You can put on the same lens of friendly curiosity when observing thoughts such as *I'm experiencing anxiety*, or *What can I do now?* or *I wish this pain would go away already!* or *Why am I feeling the way I'm feeling?* By simply looking at the chatter, you once again recognize that you are the observer; the thought is the observed. The thought is not you. By learning to merely observe our emotions, by cultivating the ability to focus and refocus on our thoughts and sensations without judgment, we can free ourselves from the second level of suffering, from the pain that we manufacture beyond the pain that is natural.

There is another important benefit to observing your emotions, beyond helping you realize that you are not your emotions. By paying attention to your emotions you recognize their true nature as impermanent and temporary rather than permanent and ever-present: This feeling, this situation, will not last forever. The idea of impermanence is central to Buddhist thought. Impermanence is about learning to see emotions as temporary. This isn't always easy to do. Sometimes, our emotions burn so strongly that we cannot see a way of cooling them off or extinguishing them altogether. And we believe that like the sun, they're here to stay—if not for a few billion years, then till death do us part. Our thoughts and sensations are so much a part of our life that they often seem to be more real than concrete objects—but when we familiarize ourselves with their true nature, we realize that they are not. Meditation is an excellent way to practice observation and become familiar with the true nature of our emotions.

Every emotion has a beginning and an end, a flow and an ebb, a rising and a falling. By observing their natural course, we realize that thoughts and sensations are not fixed structures that never go away and never change, but rather make appearances. As they come, so they go. Meditation teacher and author Matthieu Ricard writes that emotions are "just temporary and circumstantial elements of our nature."[6]

The difference between a happier individual and a depressed individual often boils down to how they perceive painful emotions: The person who is depressed experiences learned helplessness—"No matter what I do, this feeling is here to stay." The happier individual experiences painful emotions, too, but the major difference is that they know that "This, too, shall pass."

Gratitude

Lebanese-American poet Kahlil Gibran writes that we are like vessels with the capacity to experience both sorrow and joy. Each time we experience sorrow, we are carving out a little more from the inside of our vessel, which means we have a larger capacity to experience joy later. Again, when we allow ourselves to experience sorrow, anger, anxiety, and fear, we're also expanding our capacity to experience joy, love, excitement, and hope.

Cultivating pleasurable emotions is important in good times as well as in difficult ones, now or at any other time. Beyond the fact that it feels good to feel good, pleasurable emotions serve another purpose—to energize us and to broaden the possibilities we see before us. Barbara Fredrickson, psychologist and professor at the University of North Carolina, suggests, "Through experiences of positive emotions people transform themselves, becoming more creative, knowledgeable, resilient, socially integrated, and healthy individuals."[7] One of the simplest ways we can transform ourselves is by practicing gratitude. I've been keeping a gratitude journal for more than two decades—since September 19, 1999, to be exact. I started doing it because Oprah raved about it on one of her shows. And it was only a few years later, in 2003, that psychological research proved the benefits of keeping a gratitude journal. Keeping a daily or even a weekly journal can make us happier, more optimistic, and more likely to achieve our goals. It makes us kinder and more generous toward other people, as well as physically healthier.[8]

How is it that so simple an intervention can have such a powerful impact on our wellbeing? Fundamentally, good and bad things happen to everyone. At least to some extent, it's what we choose to focus on that determines how happy we are. Keeping a gratitude journal doesn't just affect those few minutes when you're thinking about and writing down the good things in your life, things you want to savor. Its reach goes much further. It's the beginning of what Robert Emmons, gratitude expert and professor of psychology at UC Davis, describes as an upward spiral of positivity: I express gratitude and then I feel better, so I'm nicer to another person and that person is nicer to me, and I feel even better. And then I do my work a little bit better, and as a result I'm gentler with my kids, I feel more fulfilled, and so on. A small positive experience can change the course of our day from being on a downward trajectory to being on an upward spiral.

Expressing gratitude is an especially useful tool when life is hard and everything around you seems gloomy. A basic premise of the science of happiness is that in every situation, you can find something to be grateful for— even if it is just being thankful for having made it through the day. Even if things are looking down, by focusing on the one or two things that are going well, you can shift the spiral upward. A single candle can light up an entire dark room.

As you keep your gratitude journal, you don't have to fall into the trap of monotony, just going through the motions of recording observations without experiencing emotion. How do you keep it interesting? First, you can find new things to focus on and express gratitude for—this world is so rich, and there is always something new we can appreciate. Second, even if you are repeating gratitudes, you can still experience freshness by visualizing and savoring. You can close your eyes and imagine whatever it is that you're grateful for. When you actively envision what you're writing about—when you activate your brain's visual cortex—you prevent yourself from going on autopilot.[9] Then, you can take a bit of time, even a few seconds, to savor and connect. Let's say I would like to express gratitude for my children, David, Shirelle, and Eliav. I start by bringing their images to mind and savoring my love for them in my heart. I connect to that love, and experience the benefit of what Barbara Fredrickson calls *heartfelt positivity*.[10] Then I write their names down in my gratitude journal. At that point, the gratitude is real. In contrast, if I just write without pausing to feel the emotion, it's not likely to be as effective.

A form of gratitude that is extremely helpful is celebrating your wins—even the small or mundane ones. Research by Harvard professor Teresa Amabile and developmental psychologist Steven Kramer suggests that taking time to reflect on one meaningful thing that you made progress on during the day makes you more productive, more creative, and increases job satisfaction.[11] The meaningful progress does not need to be major progress toward some lofty goal; any contribution to something worthwhile will do, like having a good client meeting or slightly advancing the development of a project. The "progress principle" applies to one's personal life, too. Whether it's that you got three loads of laundry done, taught your child to tie their shoes, or finally painted your living room—it all counts. Don't take for granted the good things in any area of your life—be grateful for any incremental progress you achieve.

You may be thinking, *This all sounds nice, but I don't have time to keep a gratitude journal!* Journaling need not take long—only two or three minutes a night are really all that's required. Try it, even if you only manage to make an entry once or twice a week—the effect will surprise you. In addition, if you keep a gratitude journal as a regular practice, throughout the day you'll start looking for things that you will later put in your journal. It will help you be more present. We acknowledge gratitudes as a family at least once a week, going around the dinner table with each of us sharing the things we're grateful for. I know that throughout the week my kids are collecting gratitudes, making mental notes of things they will later share with the rest of the family. This simple exercise can be a valuable ritual for you to do on your own or with others, at home or at work, in good as well as in difficult times.

Happiness Is Contagious

In the early 1990s, a number of Italian scientists isolated a single neuron in a monkey's brain. Each time the monkey brought its hand toward its mouth, this particular neuron fired. One day the scientists noticed that the neuron was firing, yet the monkey was sitting still. Initially, they thought this was some kind of glitch. But then someone realized what was going on: a scientist in the lab was eating an ice cream cone. Each time the monkey saw the scientist lift his hand, its neuron fired, reacting as if the monkey himself was doing so. They had accidentally discovered mirror neurons.[12]

Today, many research studies later, the importance of these mirror neurons is more fully understood. They are the brain cells at the very foundation of empathy and learning; it's how babies learn by imitating others. They are also, as it turns out, a key driver of emotional contagion. An emotion in one person can trigger the same emotion in another. So when we're cheerful and flash a smile or laugh out loud, we're usually boosting the mood of those around us, too.

Expressing gratitude, therefore, does not merely create an internal upward spiral, but also an external one. When we express gratitude, we feel better; when we feel better, through emotional contagion, others do, too; and when they feel better, our mirror neurons respond, and our mood improves in return. And on and on . . .

Write a Gratitude Letter

Another powerful intervention to put you and others on an upward spiral is writing a gratitude letter. Professor Martin Seligman asked his students to write a letter to a person they're grateful for. In that letter, they were to explain why they're grateful, what they appreciate about them, and then ideally read the letter to that person. Seligman says that in his decades of teaching, he had never witnessed such powerful emotions as a result of an exercise he assigned, so he conducted a research study on it with his colleagues.[13] Not surprisingly, they found that it has a real and lasting impact on the person writing the letter, on the person receiving the letter, and on the relationship.

Every year, I ask my undergraduate students to write a gratitude letter to someone. It could be to a parent, a friend, a mentor, or anyone else they appreciate. The impact of this simple exercise is quite remarkable. Here's one example: John (not his real name) was a student in my class. Even though there were close to a thousand students taking the class—this was years after my initial class of six students—I would always spot John as he entered the lecture hall. He was a big guy, a member of the Harvard football team. He would always come by himself, sit all the way in the back, and then at the end of the class walk out without a word, until one week after I assigned the gratitude letter exercise. That Tuesday, as I was packing up my notes and computer at the end of class, he approached me on the stage and asked if he could come to my office hours. I said that he could, of course. The following day in my office, he said, "Professor, this is my first time in my three years at Harvard that I've been to office hours." He had come to share with me the experience of the gratitude letter he wrote. He told me that he wrote it to his dad, and that he had gone home over the weekend to read it to him. Then he looked down, and when he looked up again, I saw that there was a small tear in his eye. He said, "After I read my dad the letter, he hugged me." John paused again, before continuing: "He hugged me for the first time since I was eight years old." He thanked me, got up, and left.

Another student, Debbie (not her real name), wrote a gratitude letter to her elementary school basketball coach. The coach had long retired, and Debbie said that reading the letter to her coach made the coach look ten years younger.

Think about who has been important to you in shaping your life. What if you wrote a gratitude letter, one letter, to thank someone who has given you a lot? Even if you write it to a person who's no longer alive, a gratitude letter still has an impact on the person writing it because you tap into that deep and authentic appreciation. So write this letter to someone who changed your life for the better. Read it to them, whether you're with them in the same enclosed space or connecting to them through technology. Or you can just email the letter. The effect that a gratitude letter has on the person writing it and on the person receiving it is powerful. Not only does it impact your emotional wellbeing, it also provides you with a sense of meaning (spiritual wellbeing) and brings you closer together (relational wellbeing). It even strengthens your immune system (physical wellbeing). If you can do this on a regular basis, even once every few months, it can really boost your wholebeing.

What if schools, as part of their curriculum, introduced the practice of a gratitude letter? What if managers, leading by example, encouraged employees to express gratitude to their colleagues and clients? Our world would be a better, kinder, happier, and healthier place.

Cultivating Hope

Finally, gratitude is not just about the past—thanking someone for what they did, or looking back on your day. It's also about the future. Psychologists Hadassah Littman-Ovadia and Dina Nir conducted a study asking people to write three things that they were looking forward to during the day.[14] They could be big things or little things—it could be a call with a friend, reading a poem, or lunch. It doesn't matter what they are, just three things they were looking forward to.

People who did this activity did not experience a spike in their pleasurable emotions. However, they *did* experience fewer painful emotions and were less pessimistic. Why is that? By having something to look forward to, which is what positive future journaling is about, we foster hope. And when we have hope, we are by definition less pessimistic. Moreover, we become more resilient, as the sadness all of us sometimes feel—unless we're psychopaths or dead—does not degenerate into depression. Once again, the difference between sadness and depression is that depression is sadness without hope.

My favorite word in English is *appreciate*, which has two meanings. To appreciate is to say thank you for something, to be grateful for it—and that's an important thing to do. The ancient Roman philosopher Cicero called gratitude the parent of all virtues. In just about every religion there's an emphasis on being grateful, being thankful, not taking things for granted. That's the first meaning of the word *appreciate*. The second meaning is to grow in value. For instance, the value of our home or of our money in the bank hopefully appreciates. The economy in healthy times appreciates. It grows.

The two meanings of the word *appreciate* are connected. Today we have the data to prove that *When you appreciate the good, the good appreciates*. When you are grateful for the good things in your life, when you do not take them for granted, the good in your life grows. Unfortunately, the opposite is also the case: When you do not appreciate the good, the good depreciates and you have less of it. Fortunately, even in difficult times, there is always something that you can be thankful for, some good in your life that you can appreciate.

Helen Keller was born with her senses intact, but at nineteen months old she suffered an illness that left her permanently deaf and blind. For five years Keller lived in a world that made no sense to her, until a teacher, Anne Sullivan, helped Keller understand the concept of words and language. This breakthrough ultimately enabled Keller to communicate and share her rich inner world with the outside world, as well as grasp the outside world and bring it in. In her essay "Three Days to See," Keller writes about what she would do if she were given three days where she could actually see and hear again.[15] This inspiring essay is a celebration of appreciation and is in itself a course in gratitude. More than any other piece of writing that I've come across, it reminds us to be grateful for what we have.

In the essay, Keller tells the story of a friend who came to visit her in Cambridge, Massachusetts, where she lived. Her friend went out for a walk in the forest, and when she came back Keller asked her what she saw. Her friend replied, "Nothing in particular." Keller responds,

> How was it possible, I asked myself, to walk for an hour through the woods and see nothing worthy of note? . . . If I can get so much pleasure from mere touch, how much more beauty must be revealed by sight. Yet, those who have eyes apparently see little. The panorama of color and action which fills the world is taken for granted. It is human, perhaps, to appreciate little that which we have and to long for that which we have not, but it is a great pity that in the world of light the gift of sight is used only as a mere convenience rather than as a means of adding fullness to life.

Helen Keller's "Three Days to See" was originally published in the *Atlantic Monthly* in 1933. Read it by yourself, read it aloud with your family, just read it. Then take a look around you. Listen, touch, taste, smell— experience the gifts the world offers using each one of your senses. There are times when it feels like we're losing out in life—and that's when our focus can benefit from gentle redirection. This essay can guide us toward taking a fresh look at what's been there all along, inside us and all around us. Why not print out this essay and put it near you on your desk or on your fridge or by your bedside? You can come back to it whenever you need a reminder to savor and appreciate all that life has to offer.

THE SPIRE CHECK-IN

Emotional Wellbeing

Go through the three steps of the SPIRE Check-In–
ascribe, describe, and prescribe–focusing on emotional
wellbeing. Begin by reflecting on the following questions:

Do you experience pleasurable emotions?

Do you embrace painful emotions?

Do you take much of what you have
in life for granted?

Do you appreciate all that you have?

Based on your reflections, determine the degree to
which you experience emotional wellbeing and then
ascribe a score from 1 to 10, with 1 being very little
or very infrequently, and 10 being very much or very
often. After ascribing a score, in writing *describe* why
you gave yourself that score. Then, *prescribe* a way
to increase your score of emotional wellbeing by just
one point at first. Examples may include introducing
a gratitude exercise daily or weekly, writing a letter
of gratitude once a week or once every other month,
keeping a journal where you can express your emotions
and allow them to flow freely, or meditating for a few
minutes each day as a way of accepting your emotions.
Keep checking in with yourself once a week.

Conclusion:
—
Moving Forward

To live happily is an inward power of the soul.
—Marcus Aurelius

Peter Drucker is considered by many to be the father of modern management studies. He was born in 1909 and died in 2005, a week short of his ninety-sixth birthday. Throughout his life Drucker traveled the world, speaking to hundreds of thousands of managers and leaders. In his later years, however, he preferred not to travel much, so instead of venturing out to speak to people, he had them come to him. Fortune 500 CEOs, political leaders, senior executive groups, they all flocked to Claremont, California, to spend a magical weekend with the grand master of management.

The way Drucker started off these weekends was by telling participants that on Monday, when they went back to their lives, to their homes and offices, he didn't want them to call him up and rave about the amazing time that they had. Rather, he wanted them to tell him what new behaviors they were introducing. He would say: "On Monday, don't tell me how great it was; tell me what you're doing differently."

Why? Because after spending more than sixty years in the business of change, Peter Drucker understood that most change efforts fail, that an insight following a weekend retreat or a self-help book, no matter how great, usually brings about nothing more than the honeymoon effect. It doesn't matter how powerful a learning experience is, most people go back to where they were before the experience.

To effectively bring about change it's not enough to have an aha moment of insight. Rather, we must apply the insight, try things out, experiment.

Here is a quick recap of the five SPIRE elements. As you read through this list and think about some of the ideas we explored in this book, ask yourself: What can I do differently in each element that can help me become happier, no matter what?

Spiritual wellbeing. We can infuse meaning and significance—a sense of purpose—in almost everything that we do. We can change the way we see our work from a job or a career to a calling. Similarly, we can find the spiritual in our everyday activities. Everything that we do, no matter how seemingly mundane, can be experienced as elevated if we bring mindful awareness to it. Just as the argument goes that we only utilize a small percentage of our brain capacity, I would argue that we only utilize a small percentage of the spiritual capacity that exists in each moment. Pay attention and be present.

Physical wellbeing. Remember, stress is not the problem. The problem is when we don't have enough recovery. We can recover on the micro-level, with a thirty-second breathing session, or the fifteen-minute break. We can experience mid-level recovery, by getting a good night's sleep or taking a day off; and we can enjoy a longer macro-level recovery, by going on a vacation (which need not involve travel). Don't forget the importance of physical exercise—even more so during stressful periods. We break down our muscles and it's good for us, it makes us stronger. That is what antifragility is about.

Intellectual wellbeing. Curiosity and openness to experience help us make the most of what life has to offer. One of the most harmful afflictions of the modern world is that deep learning has relinquished its place to superficial learning. Most people believe that they do not have enough time and that they most certainly lack the patience to deeply engage with a book or a work of art or nature. However, such deep engagement is critical for wholebeing and beyond—from succeeding in business to enjoying long-term relationships. Finally, being free to make mistakes and learn from failure is a key to growth and, in turn, a happier life.

Relational wellbeing. The number one predictor of happiness is intimate relationships. Even if we can't go out with our friends or spend as much face-to-face time as we'd like, we can still take steps to deepen our relationships. When we truly listen, when we are being listened to, when we share and open up, we feed our relationships. And we can do this virtually, too. Similarly, when we give, when we help—when we're generous and kind—we become happier and our relationships improve. Don't forget that crises are important. Lasting relationships are not ones where everything is perfect, but those in which you learn to navigate conflicts and grow together.

Emotional wellbeing. The permission to be human— allowing ourselves to experience the full range of human emotions—is always valuable, and it's certainly important in difficult times when emotions are more extreme and more complex. When we reject painful emotions, they not only intensify, but we are also inadvertently rejecting the pleasurable emotions that flow through our one emotional pipeline. One of the best ways to cultivate our emotional wellbeing is to express more gratitude—a powerful intervention that creates beneficial upward spirals in our lives.

Each element of SPIRE impacts, and is impacted by, the others. This interconnection is in itself a source of hope, because when we identify the elements of a whole, we identify the levers for change. The SPIRE Check-In can help you identify leverage points. It provides you with a summary report of sorts of your overall wholebeing, and through that it can inform your subsequent actions. I urge you to keep checking in with yourself on a regular basis. As you continue to make incremental changes to your life, you can become not only happier, but also more optimistic and hopeful for your future.

Pay It Forward

Now that you've learned about the elements of SPIRE, why not share these strategies with those whom you care about? Why not pay it forward? The basic message in the movie *Pay It Forward* is that one person can make a world of difference by capitalizing on the exponential nature of human interactions. The student, played by Haley Joel Osment, comes up with a class project to change the world by doing something good for three people, and in return asking them to pass on the good deed to three other people, who are then asked to do the same, and so on. The idea is simple, and brilliant.

Most people underestimate their ability, or the ability of a small group of people, to effect change. Research in social psychology by Charlan Nemeth, Serge Moscovici, and many others, illustrates the power of the minority—be it a small group or an individual—to make a difference and have a significant impact.[1] Along similar lines, philosopher Ralph Waldo Emerson noted, "All history is a record of the power of minorities, and of minorities of one." And as anthropologist Margaret Mead purportedly pointed out: "Never doubt that a small group of thoughtful committed citizens can change the world; indeed it's the only thing that ever has."[2]

A single individual or a small group possesses the capacity to bring about widespread, societal change because of the exponential nature of human networks. Take the example of spreading smiles: If you make three people smile, and they in turn make three different people smile, and these nine then each make three other people smile, then within twenty iterations you will reach the entire population of the world. You can radically increase your odds of influencing people the world over if you make four or ten people smile. By the same logic, if you genuinely compliment three or ten people, they are much more likely to do the same for others and accordingly spread goodness and happiness.

Happiness is contagious, and so all those whom you interact with and impact become carriers of your happiness, spreading it far and wide.[3]

Even when the going gets tough, there is always something you can do to become happier; and when you do so, you help others do the same. Remember, you are a spiritual being capable of purpose and presence. You are a physical being, a mind and body united, flowing with energy and vitality. You are an intellectual being: curious, deep, capable of learning and growing. You are a relational being, generous and kind, with the capacity to love and be loved. You are an emotional being, capable of experiencing pain and pleasure, compassion and joy.

You are whole.

Notes

Introduction

1. Taleb, N. N. (2012). *Antifragile: Things That Gain from Disorder.* Random House.

2. Calhoun, L. G. and Tedeschi, R. G. (2006). *The Handbook of Posttraumatic Growth: Research and Practice.* Routledge.

3. Gilbert, D. (2007). *Stumbling on Happiness.* Vintage Books.

4. Brickman, P., Coates, D. and Bulman, R. J. (1978). "Lottery Winners and Accident Victims: Is Happiness Relative?" *Journal of Personality and Social Psychology*, 36, 917–927.

5. Lambert, Craig (2007). "The Science of Happiness." *Harvard Magazine.*

6. Twenge, J. (2017). "With Teen Mental Health Deteriorating over Five Years, There's a Likely Culprit." *The Conversation*.

7. Lyubomirsky, S., King, L. and Diener, E. (2005). "The Benefits of Frequent Positive Affect: Does Happiness Lead to Success?" *Psychological Bulletin, 131*, 803–855.

8. Fredrickson, B. L. (2001). "The Role of Positive Emotions in Positive Psychology: The Broaden-and-Build Theory of Positive Emotions." *American Psychologist*, 56, 218–226.

9. Ibid.

10. Keller, H. (1957). *The Open Door*. Doubleday.

11. Mauss, I. B., Tamir, M., Anderson, C. L., and Savino, N. S. (2011). "Can Seeking Happiness Make People Unhappy? Paradoxical Effects of Valuing Happiness." *Emotion, 11*, 807–815.

12. Mill, J. S. (2018). *Autobiography*. Loki's Publishing.

13. Ben-Shahar, T. (2021). *Happiness Studies: An Introduction*. Palgrave Macmillan.

14. Swan, G. E., and Carmelli, D. (1996). "Curiosity and mortality in aging adults: A 5-year follow-up of the Western Collaborative Group Study." *Psychology and Aging, 11*(3), 449–453.

15. Dunn, E. and Norton, M. (2013). *Happy Money: The Science of Happier Spending*. Simon & Schuster.

16. Lyubomirsky, S., Sheldon, K. M., and Schkade, D. (2005). "Pursuing Happiness: The Architecture of Sustainable Change." *Review of General Psychology*, 9, 111.

Chapter 1

1. Wrzesniewski, A. and Dutton, J. E. (2001). "Crafting a Job: Employees as Active Crafters of Their Work." *Academy of Management Review 26*, 179–201.

2. Ibid.

3. Grant, A. (2014). *Give and Take: Why Helping Others Drives Our Success*. Penguin Books.

4. Sreechinth, C. (2018). *Thich Nhat Hanh Quotes*. UB Tech.

5. Davidson, R. J. and Harrington, A. (2001). *Visions of Compassion: Western Scientists and Tibetan Buddhists Examine Human Nature*. Oxford University Press.

6. Ibid.

7. Kabat-Zinn, J. (2013). *Full Catastrophe Living: Using the Wisdom of Your Body and Mind to Face Stress, Pain, and Illness*. Bantam Books.

8. Hanh, T. N. (1999). *The Miracle of Mindfulness: An Introduction to the Practice of Meditation* (M. Ho, trans.). Beacon Press.

9. Ricard, M. (2010). *Art of Meditation*. Atlantic Books.

10. Guthrie, C. (2008). "Mind Over Matters Through Meditation" *O, The Oprah Magazine*.

11. Goldstein, E. (2013). *The Now Effect*. Atria Books.

12. Sreechinth, C. (2018). *Thich Nhat Hanh Quotes*. UB Tech.

13. Miller, H. (1994). *Plexus: The Rosy Crucifixion II*. Grove Press.

14. Itzchakov, G. and Kluger, A. N. (2018). "The Power of Listening in Helping People Change." *Harvard Business Review*.

15. Bouskila-Yam, O. and Kluger, A. N. (2011). "Strength-Based Performance Appraisal and Goal Setting." *Human Resource Management Review*.

16. Pennebaker, J. W. (1997). *Opening Up: The Healing Power of Expressing Emotions*. The Guilford Press.

17. Csikszentmihalyi, M. (1999). "If We Are So Rich, Why Aren't We Happy?" *American Psychologist, 54,* 821–827.

18. Bennett-Goleman, T. (2002). *Emotional Alchemy: How the Mind Can Heal the Heart.* Harmony Books.

Chapter 2

1. Damasio, A. (2006). *Descartes' Error: Emotion, Reason, and the Human Brain.* Vintage Books.

2. Senge, P. M. (2006). *The Fifth Discipline: The Art and Practice of the Learning Organization.* Doubleday.

3. Zajonc, R. B., Murphy, S. T., and Inglehart, M. (1989). "Feeling and Facial Efference: Implications of the Vascular Theory of Emotion." *Psychological Review.*

4. Wiseman, R. (2013). *The As If Principle: The Radically New Approach to Changing Your Life.* Free Press.

5. Ranganathan, V. K. et al. (2003). "From Mental Power to Muscle Power—Gaining Strength by Using the Mind." *NeuroPsychologia.*

6. Elsen, A. E. et al. (2003). *Rodin's Art: The Rodin Collection of Iris & B. Gerald Cantor Center of Visual Arts at Stanford University.* Oxford University Press.

7. Lambert, Craig (2007). "The Science of Happiness." *Harvard Magazine.*

8. McGonigal, K. (2016). *The Upside of Stress: Why Stress Is Good for You, and How to Get Good at It.* Avery.

9. Loehr, J. and Schwartz, T. (2005). *The Power of Full Engagement: Managing Energy Not Time Is the Key to High Performance and Personal Renewal.* Free Press.

10. Mayo Clinic Staff (2019). "Stress Symptoms: Effects on Your Body and Behavior." *Mayo Clinic Healthy Lifestyle.*

11. Loehr, J. and Schwartz, T. (2001). "The Making of a Corporate Athlete." *Harvard Business Review.*

12. Benson, H. and Klipper, M. Z. (2000). *The Relaxation Response.* William Morrow Paperbacks.

13. Weil, A. (2001). *Breathing: The Master Key to Self Healing* (Audiobook). Sounds True.

14. Loehr, J. and Schwartz, T. (2001). "The Making of a Corporate Athlete." *Harvard Business Review.*

15. Walker, M. (2018). *Why We Sleep: Unlocking the Power of Sleep and Dreams.* Scribner.

16. Mednick, S. C. (2006). *Take a Nap! Change Your Life.* Workman Publishing.

17. Walker, M. (2018). *Why We Sleep: Unlocking the Power of Sleep and Dreams.* Scribner.

18. Ibid.

19. Ibid.

20. Ibid.

21. Rand Corporation (2016). "Lack of Sleep Costing U.S. Economy Up to $411 Billion a Year" (press release). rand.org/news/press/2016/11/30 (accessed October 27, 2020).

22. Mednick, S. C. (2006). *Take a Nap! Change Your Life*. Workman Publishing.

23. Carino, M. M. (2019). "American Workers Can Suffer Vacation Guilt… If They Take Vacations at All." *Marketplace*. zmarketplace.org/2019/07/12/ american-workers-vacation-guilt (accessed November 27, 2020).

24. Loehr, J. and Schwartz, T. (2005). *The Power of Full Engagement: Managing Energy, Not Time, Is the Key to High Performance and Personal Renewal*. Free Press.

25. Ibid.

26. Ratey, J. J. (2013). *Spark: The Revolutionary New Science of Exercise and the Brain*. Little, Brown and Company.

27. Callaghan, P. (2004). "Exercise: A Neglected Intervention in Mental Health Care?" *Journal of Psychiatric and Mental Health Nursing.*

28. Ratey, J. J. (2013). *Spark: The Revolutionary New Science of Exercise and the Brain.* Little, Brown and Company.

29. Callaghan, P. (2004). "Exercise: A Neglected Intervention in Mental Health Care?" *Journal of Psychiatric and Mental Health Nursing.*

30. Van der Ploeg H.P. et al. (2012). "Sitting Time and All-Cause Mortality Risk in 222 497 Australian Adults." *Archives of Internal Medicine,* 172, 494–500.

31. Ratey, J. J. (2013). *Spark: The Revolutionary New Science of Exercise and the Brain.* Little, Brown and Company.

32. Ibid.

33. Buettner, D. (2012). *The Blue Zones: 9 Lessons for Living Longer from the People Who've Lived the Longest.* National Geographic.

34. Steel, P. (2012). *The Procrastination Equation: How to Stop Putting Things Off and Start Getting Stuff Done.* Harper Perennial.

35. Cuddy, A. (2018). *Presence: Bringing Your Boldest Self to Your Biggest Challenges.* Little, Brown and Company.

Chapter 3

1. Csikszentmihalyi, M. (2014). *Applications of Flow in Human Development and Education: The Collected Works of Mihaly Csikszentmihalyi.* Springer.

2. Kashdan, T. B. (2010). *Curiosity: The Missing Ingredient to a Fulfilling Life.* Harper Perennial.

3. Bem, D. J. (1967). "Self-perception: An Alternative Interpretation of Cognitive Dissonance Phenomena." *Psychological Review*, 74, 183–200.

4. Lakkakula, A. (2010). "Repeated Taste Exposure Increases Liking for Vegetables by Low-income Elementary School Children." *Appetite*, 226–31.

5. Swan, G. E. and Carmelli, D. (1996). "Curiosity and mortality in aging adults: A 5-year follow-up of the Western Collaborative Group Study." *Psychology and Aging, 11*(3), 449–453.

6. Cooperrider, D. L. and Whitney, D. (2005). *Appreciative Inquiry: A Positive Revolution in Change.* Berrett-Koehler Publishers.

7. Suzuki, S. (2020). *Zen Mind, Beginner's Mind: Informal Talks on Zen Meditation and Practice.* Shambhala.

8. Langer, E. J. (2014). *Mindfulness: 25th Anniversary Edition.* Da Capo Lifelong Books.

9. Simonton, D. (1999). *Origins of Genius: Darwinian Perspectives on Creativity.* Oxford University Press.

10. Dweck, C. (2005). *Mindset: The New Psychology of Success.* Ballantine Books.

11. Roosevelt, T. "Citizenship in a Republic: The Man in the Arena." Leadership Now. leadershipnow.com/tr-citizenship.html (accessed October 27, 2020).

12. Neff, K. (2011). *Self-Compassion: The Proven Power of Being Kind to Yourself.* William Morrow.

13. Dweck, C. (2005). *Mindset: The New Psychology of Success.* Ballantine Books.

14. Edmondson, A. (1999). "Psychological Safety and Learning Behavior in Work Teams." *Administrative Science Quarterly 44,* 350.

15. Delizonna, L. (2017). "High Performing Teams Need Psychological Safety. Here's How to Create It." *Harvard Business Review.*

16. Kelly, A. (2017). "James Burke: The Johnson & Johnson CEO Who Earned a Presidential Medal of Freedom." jnj.com (Johnson & Johnson website). jnj.com/our-heritage/james-burke-johnson-johnson-ceo-who-earned-presidential-medal-of-freedom (accessed November 25, 2020).

17. Rilke, R. M. (1993). *Letters to a Young Poet*. W. W. Norton & Company.

Chapter 4

1. Waldinger, R. (2015). "What Makes a Good Life? Lessons from the Longest Study on Happiness." ted.com. https://www.ted.com/talks/robert_waldinger_what_makes_a_good_life_lessons_from_the_longest_study_on_happiness (accessed October 27, 2020).

2. Helliwell, J., Layard, R. and Sachs, J. (2019). *World Happiness Report*. https://worldhappiness.report/ed/2019/ (accessed August 23, 2019).

3. Klinenberg, E. (2013). *Going Solo: The Extraordinary Rise and Surprising Appeal of Living Alone*. Penguin Books.

4. Twenge, J. (2017). "With Teen Mental Health Deteriorating over Five Years, There's a Likely Culprit." *The Conversation*.

5. Konrath, S. H., O'Brien, E. H. and Hsing, C. (2010). "Changes in Dispositional Empathy in American College Students Over Time: A Meta-Analysis." *Personality and Social Psychology Review, 15*, 180–198.

6. Hoffman, M. L. (2001). *Empathy and Moral Development: Implications for Caring and Justice*. Cambridge University Press.

7. Dunn, E. and Norton, M. (2013). *Happy Money: The Science of Happier Spending.* Simon & Schuster.

8. Grant, A. (2014). *Give and Take: Why Helping Others Drives Our Success.* Penguin Books.

9. Goleman, D. (2004). *Destructive Emotions: How Can We Overcome Them?* Bantam Books.

10. Ibid.

11. Winnicott, D. W. (2002). *Winnicott on the Child.* Da Capo Lifelong Books.

12. Luthar, S. S. and Becker, B. E. (2002). "Privileged but pressured? A study of affluent youth." *Child Development, 73*(5), 1593–1610.

13. Montessori, M. (2009). *The Absorbent Mind.* BN Publishing.

14. Christensen, C. (2012). "The School of Life." *Harvard Business School Alumni Online.* alumni.hbs.edu/stories/Pages/story-bulletin.aspx?num=814 (accessed November 27, 2020).

15. Emerson, R. W. (1909). *The Works of Ralph Waldo Emerson: Letters and Social Aims.* Fireside Edition.

16. Kuhn, R. (2018). "The Power of Listening: Lending an Ear to the Partner During Dyadic Coping Conversations." *Journal of Family Psychology,* 32, 762–772.

Chapter 5

1. Wegner, D. M. (1994). *White Bears and Other Unwanted Thoughts: Suppression, Obsession, and the Psychology of Mental Control.* The Guilford Press.

2. Marcin, A. (2017). *9 Ways Crying May Benefit Your Health. Healthline.* healthline.com/health/benefits-of-crying (accessed November 27, 2020).

3. Straker, G. and Winship, J. (2019). *The Talking Cure: Normal People, Their Hidden Struggles and the Life-Changing Power of Therapy.* Macmillan Australia.

4. Pennebaker, J. W. (1997). *Opening Up: The Healing Power of Expressing Emotions.* The Guilford Press.

5. Williams, M., et al. (2007). *The Mindful Way Through Depression: Freeing Yourself from Chronic Unhappiness.* The Guilford Press.

6. Ricard, M. (2010). *Art of Meditation.* Atlantic Books.

7. Fredrickson, B. L. (2001). "The Role of Positive Emotions in Positive Psychology: The Broaden-and-Build Theory of Positive Emotions." *American Psychologist*, 56, 218–226.

8. Emmons, R. (2008). *Thanks: How Practicing Gratitude Can Make You Happier.* Mariner Books.

9. Kosslyn, S. M., Thompson, W. L and Ganis, G. (2006). *The Case for Mental Imagery*. Oxford University Press.

10. Fredrickson, B. L. (2001). "The Role of Positive Emotions in Positive Psychology: The Broaden-and-Build Theory of Positive Emotions." *American Psychologist*, 56, 218-226.

11. Amabile, T. and Kramer, S. (2011). *Progress Principle: Using Small Wins to Ignite Joy, Engagement, and Creativity at Work*. Harvard Business Review Press.

12. Ferrari, P. F., and Rizzolatti, G. (2014). "Mirror Neuron Research: The Past and the Future." *Philosophical Transactions of the Royal Society of London. Series B, Biological Sciences*, 369 (1644).

13. Seligman, M. E. P., Steen, T. A., Park, N. and Peterson, C. (2005). "Positive Psychology Progress: Empirical Validation of Interventions." *American Psychologist*, 60, 410–421.

14. Littman-Ovadia, H. and Nir, D. (2013). "Looking Forward to Tomorrow: The Buffering Effect of a Daily Optimism Intervention." *Journal of Positive Psychology*, 9(2):122–136.

15. Keller, H. (1933). "Three Days to See." *Atlantic Monthly*. afb.org/about-afb/history/helen-keller/books-essays-speeches/senses/three-days-see-published-atlantic (accessed November 27, 2020).

Conclusion

1. Nemeth, C. (1974). *Social Psychology: Classic and Contemporary Integrations (7th Ed.)*. Rand McNally.

2. Sommers, F. (1984). *Curing Nuclear Madness*. Methuen.

3. Christakis, N. A. and Fowler, J. H. (2009). *Connected: The Surprising Power of Our Social Networks and How They Shape Our Lives*. Little, Brown and Company.

Acknowledgments

Whether we experience these challenging times as the spring of hope or the winter of despair largely depends on the people in our lives. In this respect I have been blessed.

There are a few colleagues and friends without whom I would not have written this book. First, Katie McHugh Malm, whose words and wisdom are intimately intertwined throughout the book. Batya Rosenblum from The Experiment and Rafe Sagalyn of the Sagalyn Agency came up with the idea for writing this book, and continued to provide their invaluable insights throughout the process.

My fellow journeyers at the Happiness Studies Academy are working tirelessly, around the clock, helping thousands of students the world over navigate through difficult times, spreading happiness and goodness and kindness.

Angus Ridgway, my business partner and dear friend, teaches me each time we interact what it means to be a leader, when sailing is smooth and when the seas are rough.

And though since the breakout of COVID-19 I have been physically distant from my parents, siblings, and their families, their care and support are ever growing. And though since the breakout of COVID-19 I have been physically closer to my wife and children, my love for them is ever growing.

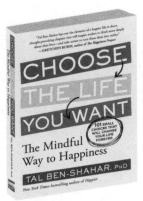
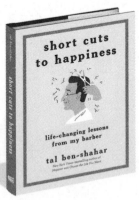

Sign up for a Certificate in Happiness Studies

CREATED AND DELIVERED
BY DR. TAL BEN-SHAHAR

———

The Certificate in Happiness Studies is a yearlong online academic course that provides the knowledge and tools to generate happiness on the individual, interpersonal, organizational, and national levels.

Includes lifetime access to:

- 40 hours of prerecorded lectures
- Live webinars
- Meditations, exercises, journaling, reading, and video content
- Vibrant and supportive international community

"This program has changed the way I see life . . . taught me the real meaning of success."
—Isabel Castro

10% off with the code: **HAPPIER**

———

For more information visit:
happinessstudies.academy/CiHS

About the Author

The author of multiple international bestselling books, TAL BEN-SHAHAR, PhD, taught two of the largest classes in Harvard University's history, "Positive Psychology" and "The Psychology of Leadership." He is the cofounder and chief learning officer of the Happiness Studies Academy and Potentialife.

talbenshahar.com